FROM BURNOUT
TO BEST LIFE

*How to take charge of your
health & happiness*

LISA HAMMETT

Published by

AVIVA
PUBLISHING
New York

From Burnout to Best Life — How to Take Charge of Your Health & Happiness
Copyright © 2022 Lisa Hammett

Published by:
Aviva Publishing
Lake Placid, NY
https://avivapubs.com

Every attempt has been made to properly source all quotes.

All inquiries:
Lisa Hammett Success Coach
www.lisahammett.com
info@lisahammett.com

ISBN: 978-1-66786-650-5 (Paperback)
ISBN: 978-1-63618-234-6 (ebook)
Library of Congress Control Number: 2022913799

Editor: Jane Maulucci, The Reactive Voice
Front cover design: Yael Halpern, YHalpern Designs
Book layout design: Michelle VanGeest
Cover art: Kim Guthrie, Kim Guthrie Art
Author photo: Lee Ann Baker, LAB Photography

First printing edition 2022
Printed in the United States of America

10 9 8 7 6 5 4 3 2 1

TABLE OF CONTENTS

FOREWORD

If you've ever experienced burnout, it's like hitting a wall. You're done! You are mentally and physically wiped out. You've lost your capacity to see beyond your present situation. Life is bleak.

This burnout was me in 2005 when I left the corporate retailing world. I was exhausted from 80-hour workweeks. I was forced into a position where I found no passion or purpose, only monotony and dissatisfaction. I was at my heaviest weight, and I felt terrible. My relationship with my husband was suffering. My joints and feet hurt, I hated the way I looked, and at 40 years old, I had hit rock bottom.

I could lose my spouse, chronic health problems were looming in front of me, and I could become the worst version of myself. I was so close. That was the tipping point. I knew I had to make serious changes.

And I did, and now I want to guide you back from the edge of burnout to leading your best life.

Once upon a time...

I considered a career as an oceanographer since I loved math, science, and the ocean. However, when I realized it required eight years of post-graduate work with an annual starting salary of $20K, I changed to computer engineering. Unfortunately, that lasted one semester due to my nemesis, calculus. The course handed me my first D, a difficult pill to swallow, as I was accustomed to a 4.0 GPA.

I made the change to business administration, with an emphasis on marketing. I had always been intrigued by marketing and advertising. When I graduated, I envisioned a long career with Procter & Gamble or Johnson & Johnson. However, neither company granted me an interview.

Three months post-graduation, and still no job prospect in sight, I was beyond discouraged.

1

So, when a local department store chain offered me an entry-level management position, I jumped at the opportunity. Thus began a 26-year love/hate relationship in the retail industry.

I loved the fast-paced, ever-changing environment. It was stimulating, and it challenged me. I was not intimidated by hard work. I was quickly promoted, and I worked my way up in store management, eventually becoming a store manager, operations manager; then seeking change, I made the shift into buying and eventually into planning.

In April of 2002, my husband and I moved from the California Bay Area to Plano, Texas. We had never lived outside of California, but we were both fed up with the cost of living and needed a change. Plus, I was offered a terrific opportunity with a major retailer in the Dallas-Fort Worth area, so I signed a two-year contract, thinking we would be in Texas for a couple of years and then move elsewhere. That was over 20 years ago.

In 2003, I attended my first direct selling home party hosted by one of my neighbors. She introduced me to Southern Living at HOME (SLAH), a rapidly growing company featuring a beautiful line of home décor. I immediately fell in love with the products, wanting everything in the catalog. While I watched the consultant deliver her presentation, I thought: "I can do that! How fun would that be?"

I tucked that thought away, decided to book a party, and over the next year, I became a loyal purchaser of SLAH. Periodically, I'd think about becoming a consultant but never took it seriously, as my work schedule was hectic. I barely had time for anything else.

We were on vacation in California about six months later, visiting family and friends. The wife of one of my best friends was a SLAH Director, and she shared the latest catalog with me. When I commented that I loved everything in the catalog, she suggested that I become a consultant. Of course, I objected and told her I had no time. But, being the great Director that she was, she empathized with my situation and shared that by becoming a consultant, I could earn back what I spent on product purchases.

My husband, overhearing our conversation, quickly chimed in, noting that if I could offset my purchases, it would be a huge win! He also mentioned that it would be a fun outlet for me since I was working all the time. "I don't have time for this!" was my first thought. However, after further encouragement, I took the plunge.

I worked my business alongside my corporate job. It was challenging, but I loved it! I loved the social interaction. Selling the product was easy. Finally, I began to see how I could make substantial income in my direct sales business.

Fast forward to September 2005 and my tipping point. I took a leap of faith, left the corporate world, and started an amazing 16-year journey in the direct selling/network marketing industry. I earned many incentive trips to five-star resorts that I would never have visited otherwise. I joined the industry because of the product. I stayed in the industry for the relationships and personal growth. Some of my closest friendships have formed from relationships with fellow consultants and clients. I have learned so much about myself.

When I left my corporate career and began my new path in direct sales, I also started my second health and wellness journey. My first weight loss experience was in California, where I lost 45 pounds and kept it off for three years. However, when we moved to Texas, my old eating habits resurfaced. I was using food as a stress management coping method. To conquer my stress and weight gain, I rejoined my membership with one of the largest global wellness companies and lost 65 pounds. I became a service provider and have been one ever since. For me, there is no greater pleasure than helping others find balance by overcoming mindset challenges, creating sustainable healthy habits, and building confidence.

In 2020 the world changed forever. By May of 2020, I faced the decision of what to do for the rest of my life. The direct sales company I was working for at that time decided to close its doors. I loved wellness coaching but needed to make more money. My Christian faith led me to pray for direction.

For years, my husband had encouraged me to start my own business. I contemplated incorporating my retail and marketing experience with my current coaching into a business model. Then a friend who had been struggling with COVID weight gain and a stressful job asked if I would coach her. "Why not?" I thought. It would pair nicely with what I was already doing. I figured it was a one-off experience, never thinking it would turn into a business. However, my first client quickly turned into four clients, two of whom signed six-month contracts. My success coaching business was born.

In July of 2021, I joined an International Coaching Program through HPC — High Performing Coach. In the three-month intensive "Launch" program, I had several personal breakthroughs that have helped me in my personal development, provided valuable insight, and enabled me to serve my clients better. Leaning into my corporate, direct selling, and coaching experience, I guide stressed and burned-out business executives and owners to create balance in their lives and become healthy.

Managing stress plays an integral part in wellness, but so does identifying triggers, shifting mindset, and building sustainable healthy habits. Specific, realistic goal setting and weekly accountability make goal achievement possible.

And that's my journey to where I am today. Where are you in your life journey? Are you burned out and stressed, feeling stuck in a job that lacks fulfillment and purpose? You may have a strong desire to begin a new career and possibly open your own business but don't know where to start. If this resonates with you, I hope you find valuable insight in this book.

I am cheering you on in your journey to greatness!

Lisa Hammett

SECTION I

Getting Started

"Dream higher than the sky
and deeper than the ocean."

Rumi, Persian poet & scholar

CHAPTER 1

CREATE A LASER-FOCUSED VISION

Stop for one minute and think: If you could have anything in life, what would it be? Financial freedom, fulfilling relationships, your dream job, excellent health, or maybe the perfect home or car? You get to choose your dream.

If you don't have what you most desire, what's stopping you? Do you feel you're not good enough or deserving enough? Maybe you think these desires are not reality, at least for most people. What if I told you, you could have anything you want in life?

Would it require commitment and effort on your part? Absolutely! Will there be times when you're discouraged and want to quit? Yes! However, if you knew you could not fail, would you go for it? Of course, you would. And you can!

I love helping others envision their best life and making it their reality. Believing a better life is possible is the first step. You may not know how you'll get there, but you believe it can happen.

Getting started involves releasing limiting beliefs that you're not good enough or deserving enough to have what you desire. Often, these beliefs are formed early in life from our experiences and relationships. What we learned from our parents, teachers, and other role models creates our belief system. These thoughts can become locked in our subconscious, making them unrecognizable. Eventually, they bubble up and impact our behavior.

Consider Suzi. She has a strong desire to lose weight but has never been successful because she has the limiting belief that she can never lose weight. She developed this mindset as a child when her parents told her she was chubby like all her other family members. It was in their genes. Therefore, they would never be thin like regular people.

Changing your mindset is where a coach can be particularly helpful. A coach will recognize the belief system driving the behavior and create a safe space for reflection. Purposeful reflection can be the most difficult part of the journey, as it may bring up painful feelings. However, it is also the most liberating.

> Getting started involves releasing limiting beliefs that you're not good enough or deserving enough to have what you desire.

In July of 2021, I joined a global coaching program through HPC — High Performing Coach. During the program, I had several personal breakthroughs about myself. What I discovered was a fear of failure. I had always considered myself a confident person. Outwardly I appeared very confident. I hid my limiting belief in my subconscious. Investing in HPC was the first step in releasing this belief, although I did not know it at the time. I had never invested this much money in my self-development before.

The second step was having a skilled coach recognize how my behavior was masking something deeper. What manifested as a perfectionistic, people-pleasing mindset was actually a fear of failure. Once I became aware of this mindset, I moved past it, created my vision for the future, and took the necessary action steps.

It all starts with the belief that positive change is possible. Once the belief is there, it's time to create the vision. By definition, a vision is the ability to think about or plan the future with imagination or wisdom.

When you have created a strong vision, you have a crystal-clear picture of the future you desire. You may not know how you'll get there, but you believe that your future is possible. For a vision to come to fruition, you must have specific goals that drive your actions. Think of your "Why" as your purpose for achieving your vision. We'll discuss your "Why" in Chapter 2.

Your emotions bring life to your vision. Imagine how you will feel when you are healthy and fit. What is your energy level? Then, picture the physical things you'll be able to do.

If you are envisioning your dream job, imagine your perfect workday. Picture what you are doing and experience how it makes you feel. Imagine how you present yourself and how others respond to you. How do you feel? Are you calm and confident or excited and energized?

When I work with clients, we spend time developing a clear vision starting with a process I call brain dumping. Brain dumping involves writing down everything that comes to mind in a journal, on a whiteboard, or on sticky notes making it easy to categorize thoughts on a poster board. Once the ideas start to take shape, meditative visualization exercises can help attach feelings to the vision.

For Suzi, her brain dump may be divided into columns that include:
- How will I feel when I lose weight?
- What will I be able to do when I lose weight?

Suzi will take her responses from the brain dump and sort them to get a clearer vision and the emotion of her weight-loss goal.

How will I feel?	*What will I be able to do?*
• Increased confidence	• Travel internationally
• More energy	• Play with my grandkids
• Healthier mind and body	• Quality sleep
• Fewer aches and pains	• Drop medication

VISION BOARD

Creating a vision board is another way to develop a crystal-clear vision. By definition, a vision board is a collage of drawings and graphics infused with words and phrases that represent your vision for your best life. It's a reminder of what truly matters to you and incorporates your deepest desires.

Vision boards are powerful tools for developing a focus on what is most important to you. In addition, it is empowering since you decide what goes on your vision board.

By looking at your vision board, your brain starts to believe your vision is possible. In addition, the vision board focuses your thoughts on positive transformation and goal achievement. These beliefs drive your behavior and motivate you when you face a setback or get stuck.

You can create a vision board on your own or make it a collaborative art project with a friend. Then you can hold each other accountable for achieving the desires on the vision board.

Consider your vision board as a visual road map to your best life, and to get there, you need to pay attention to your map. Vision boards work when they are readily visible. Putting your vision board in a drawer for occasional review will not work. It must be viewed multiple times throughout the day.

Ideas for a vision board:
- Images of your bucket-list destination
- A picture of your dream house or car
- Images of bucket-list activities
- The title of your first book
- A picture of yourself at your healthy weight
- Quotes that motivate and inspire you
- Pictures of friends, family, and others you want in your life
- An image of your first paycheck when you've reached your financial goal

There is no rule on how you create your vision board. You can do it virtually (think screen-saver on your computer, tablet, or phone) or with art supplies. If you're creating a physical board, you might consider framing it for preservation.

What you'll need to create your physical vision board:
❑ Poster board or thick construction paper
❑ Scissors
❑ Glue stick
❑ Magazines
❑ Your favorite quotes
❑ Stickers, ribbon, embellishments
❑ Colored markers

Allow yourself plenty of time to create your vision board. You don't have to complete it in one sitting. Instead, walk away from it, clear your brain, and then come back to it with increased energy. In the end, you will have a vision board that reflects your values and goals, providing you with guidance, inspiration, and excitement as you work toward your desires.

Reflection questions:

1) How will having a laser-focused vision help you achieve what you want in life?

2) Schedule the date, time, and place that you will create your vision board. Remember, you can do it solo or with others for added accountability.

3) Snap a picture of your vision board and keep it handy on your phone.

_____

_____

_____

_____

_____

CHAPTER 2

DETERMINE YOUR WHY

Have you ever taken the time to really think about *WHY* you want to achieve specific goals in life? I'm not referring to superficial reasons… appearance, improved health, more money, etc. There is nothing wrong with these reasons, which may be important goals. However, they are not tied to your emotions.

Emotions involve feelings, which bring goals to life. Which option sounds better?

I want to lose weight for my health.

OR

I want to lose weight and be healthy so I am more confident, a positive role model for my children, and will have the opportunity to actively participate in my grandchildren's lives as I age.

The second version is more specific and attaches your emotions to the outcome.

When it comes to goal achievement, it's important to have a strong *"Why."* A *"Why"* statement is tied to your skills, expertise, purpose, values, and passion. It's the reason why you want to make positive changes in your life.

Your *"Why"* is the motivating component behind your vision. In the above example, health and family may be your core values. Your passion is spending quality time with your grandkids.

By simply stating, *"I want to lose weight for my health,"* you are not inspired or motivated. Instead, your strong "Why" pushes you through your challenges because you have tied your emotions to your outcome.

My *"Why"* is to maintain a healthy weight to prevent surgeries, avoid medication, and comfortably travel the world with my husband when we retire. Health is one of my core values. I've had one knee replacement and do not wish to have another. That surgery was a difficult experience with a long, painful healing process.

> **Your "Why" is the motivating component behind your vision.**

Sharing your *"Why"* with a friend, family member, colleague, mentor, or coach will hold you accountable. In addition, regular progress check-ins will provide further accountability.

If you don't have a *"Why"* it's time for another brain dump. Take a piece of paper and create three columns labeled: Values, Passions, and Strengths/Skills.

Core **Values** are those things that you value most in life. You may have different values for your personal and professional lives. Some examples include:

• Family	• Authenticity
• Health	• Vulnerability
• Faith	• Tenacity
• Honesty	• Influence
• Integrity	• Knowledge

Passions are those things that create a fire in your belly. Passions drive you to take action. Examples include:

• Serving others	• Music
• Learning about other cultures	• Sports
• Staying fit and healthy	• Art
• Personal growth and development	• Gardening

Strengths/Skills are those things that come naturally to you or you have become skilled at. Examples include:

• Active listening	• Painting
• Organization	• Communication
• Dancing	• Planning
• Writing	• Professional expertise
• Public speaking	• Singing/songwriting
• Compassion	• Teaching

Once you've created your lists, you'll start to see commonalities. Your *"Why"* is a blending of each of your columns. Your *"Why"* is closely linked to your goals. We'll discuss how to set achievable goals in the next chapter.

Reflection questions:

1) What are your core values?

2) What are your passions?

3) What are your strengths/skills?

4) How will you incorporate your values, passions, and skills into a *"Why"*?

_____

_____

_____

_____

ESTABLISH GOALS THA. JTICK

One of the top New Year's Resolutions, year after year, is getting healthy and fit. Most often, it involves losing weight. On January 1st, countless individuals declare the new year will be the year they not only lose weight but keep it off. They flock to gyms and weight loss centers. Motivation runs high for the first couple of weeks, then begins to wane.

According to recent New Year's Resolution statistics, 25 percent of those who make resolutions drop off after one week. After two weeks, the number increases to 29 percent. By the end of January, drop-offs have increased to 36 percent. After six months, drop-offs reach 54 percent. So why is it that New Year's Resolutions fail for the majority?

Good intentions alone will not produce results; a sound plan and specific action must follow intention. A great place to start is using the SMART Goal method.

SMART Goals
S pecific
M easurable
A chievable
R elevant
T ime-Bound

SPECIFIC

actions to be specific, they must include the following:

- What you are going to do
- When you are going to do it
- How often you will do it
- Who you will do it with

For example, stating that you'll lose weight by eating healthy and going to the gym sets the intention but does not provide a road map to get there.

An example of **specific** goals would be:

- *I will incorporate one to two servings of fruits and vegetables with every meal and snack.*
- *I will measure my food before I eat it, to ensure I am eating the correct portion size.*

MEASURABLE

Measurable goals include specifics such as day, time, how much, and for how long.

- *I will work out at the gym on Monday, Wednesday, and Friday.*
- *I will work out first thing in the morning for 45 minutes.*
- *I will spend 15 minutes strength training and 30 minutes riding the recumbent bike.*

ACHIEVABLE

Achievable goals are truly doable. They involve some effort, but it's highly probable they'll be achieved. Realistic goals build momentum. As humans, we want instant gratification. Feeling successful gives us gratification. When goals are unrealistic, it's easy to lose motivation and give up.

For example, expecting to lose 20 pounds in one month is not realistic. That's an average of five pounds per week. A healthy, **realistic** weight loss goal is to lose an average of one to two pounds per week. Some weeks it may be less. Some weeks it may be more. This is an average over a four-week period. Expecting to lose four to give pounds in one month is achievable.

- *I will lose at least four pounds each month.*
- *I will drink a glass of water as soon as I wake up.*

RELEVANT

Relevant goals are crucial for sustainability. A relevant goal is something you want to do versus something you feel you should do. For example, have you ever had a gym membership but didn't go to the gym consistently or at all?

You may come up with a million reasons why you don't go to the gym. If you **wanted** to go to the gym, you would make a point of going. Feeling that you **should** do something is not motivating.

It's similar to your mother telling you to eat your vegetables or clean your room when you were a child. Neither was motivating. If your mother offered that you could have dessert if you finished your vegetables, that might have been a motivator. The bottom line, no one enjoys being told what to do. Feeling that you *should* do something is your mind's way of telling you what to do. You will be more successful if you choose what you **want** to do.

- *I will walk with a friend each Saturday morning.*
- *I will take a five-minute meditation break after lunch.*

TIME-BOUND

Setting a time limit to complete your goal creates accountability. Just saying you'll start walking this week provides no accountability or sense of urgency. Before you know it, the week has gone by, and you haven't walked at all. Instead set a clear expectation:

I'll walk for 30 minutes on Tuesday and Thursday morning, before work.

To achieve your goals you must have a motivating component. That's where a strong *"Why"* comes into play. As discussed in the previous chapter, when our *"Why"* is aligned with our values, passions, and strengths, it will inspire us to take positive action.

Goals often fail because the mindset is not there.

How do Olympians win gold medals? They wake up every day with a "winner's mindset." They visualize the win, how they will feel, and how the crowd will react. They have a clear mental picture of success.

The key to successful visualization is to tie it to an emotion and believe that goal achievement is possible. See yourself achieving your goal. What will your life be like? Who will you surround yourself with? How will others perceive you? Now imagine

> **Good intentions alone will not produce results; a sound plan and specific action must follow intention.**

how you will physically and emotionally feel. Paint a clear mental picture. Close your eyes, and spend several minutes each morning, focusing on it.

In Section II, we'll take a deeper dive into a winning mindset.

If you don't believe your goals are achievable, you will not be successful. If you desire to lose weight, but your mind is telling you, "I'll never lose weight. I've never been successful," you will not lose weight.

Our mindset forms our belief system, which drives our behavior. There must be a belief that reaching the goal is possible. Many individuals struggle with fear of success, and that mindset sabotages the best of intentions. Creating a positive, growth-focused mindset takes work.

When I work with clients, we delve into the emotions that are driving their mindset and behavior before we set goals and create an action plan. My clients often discover they have limiting beliefs, developed from childhood, that are sabotaging their efforts to be successful. Once these beliefs are recognized and accepted as untruths, they can be replaced with helpful, encouraging thoughts that will drive positive behavior change.

When contemplating what you'd like to accomplish at any time, ask yourself these questions:	
What progress have I made in my life journey? (i.e., health & wellness, career, family, finances)	How has that benefited me? How does that make me feel?
Who are the people in my life who matter most?	How has their support impacted my journey?
What have I learned?	What new habits have I created? How have these improved my life?
What obstacles have I overcome?	How is my life different as a result?
What experiences or opportunities have I taken advantage of that have had an impact on my life today?	What have I done that has made a difference in the lives of others?

Spending time reflecting on positive change and those things you've accomplished is a powerful exercise. It's not about bragging and comparing yourself to others. It's about acknowledging your own successes and channeling that understanding into creating a better version of yourself. You'll be surprised at the impact counting your wins has on your mood and motivation.

Reflection questions:

1) How have you been successful this year? This month? This week?

2) What has been your biggest challenge?

3) What SMART Goal will you set this week?

_____

_____

_____

_____

_____

CHAPTER 4

BUILD SUSTAINABLE HABITS

We experience many changes during our lifetimes that add joy, sorrow, and extra stress. For example, losing a loved one, starting a new job, moving to a different city, getting married, or starting a family are significant life changes that impact behavior. When our environments change our behaviors change.

The pandemic in 2020 was a perfect example of this. Families had to adjust to working from home. Children moved to virtual learning. For many individuals, these changes made it difficult to maintain healthy habits. Going to the gym was no longer an option and lifestyles became sedentary. Often when one habit changes, it impacts other habits. Habits are the action steps for goal achievement and maintenance. Therefore, when habits are impacted, goal achievement and maintenance are impacted. To further understand the connection between habits and motivation, it's necessary to have an understanding of how habits are formed.

BUST A MYTH — 21 DAYS TO CHANGE A HABIT

For some people, this might be the case. However, there is insufficient substantiated evidence to support that all habits are formed in 21 days. Consider smoking as an example. If the desire is to quit smoking, the

21-day rule would imply that an individual can quit smoking in 21 days. You may know of someone who quit smoking cold turkey. They decided one morning to quit, and they did. For others, it may take months, even years, to quit smoking. Some individuals never do.

There are three steps to habit formation; Cue, Behavior, and Reward. Think about a triangle. At the top point of the triangle, the first step is the **Cue** or trigger. The cue is the reminder to do the behavior. An example would be setting the alarm on your phone to remind yourself to do a healthy task like getting up and moving for five minutes or drinking water.

The second component in the triangle, at the bottom right corner, is the **Behavior** or habit you wish to form. In this example, the behavior would be getting up and moving or drinking a glass of water.

The third component in habit formation, at the bottom left corner of the HABIT triangle, is the **Reward**. The reward is the benefit of doing the habit. Potential rewards include losing or maintaining weight, improved overall health, and clearer skin in this example. Positive habits are formed when these three components are all in place.

In his book, *Atomic Habits*, best-selling author James Clear states four rules that make the habit formation process easier and more enjoyable.

1) **Make your habit obvious** — Create a visual cue that spurs you to take action. The easier it is to see something that reminds you to take action, the more likely it is to maintain the activity. For example, put your favorite water glass on the counter by the coffee pot. When you see the glass, you are triggered to drink water before making your coffee.

2) **Make your habit attractive** — When the habit is appealing, you are more motivated to take action. For example, tap water may not appeal to you, but adding a squeeze of fresh lemon or lime may make it much more desirable.

3) **Make your habit easy** — Small, realistic actions that require less friction are more likely to turn into habits—having

a distinctive water glass next to the faucet has set you up for success to drink more water.

4) **Make your habit satisfying** — When you feel accomplished and successful after performing an action, you are more likely to stick with it long-term. For example, making your bed every morning gives you a feeling of accomplishment to start your day.

When forming habits, habit-stacking can be very effective. Habit-stacking is a technique where a new habit is attached to something you're already doing, which becomes the reward.

For example, let's assume you wish to drink more water throughout the day. Having your favorite water glass by the coffee pot is your **cue** to drink a glass of water. Drinking the water is the **behavior** (habit) you wish to adopt. The **reward** is having your cup of coffee. You are attaching this new habit to your current practice of drinking a cup of coffee first thing in the morning.

> Habits are the action steps for goal achievement and maintenance.

Neuroscientists have found a part of our brain called basal ganglia, which is crucial for habit formation. Our brains contain neural pathways, a series of connected nerves, which send electrical impulses through the body. Think of neural pathways as the wiring in our brain. When a particular behavior occurs, a neural pathway is formed.

The more often the behavior occurs, the stronger the pathway becomes. Once a neural pathway for a habit is established in our brain, it never goes away. This is great news, as the thinking part of the brain can concentrate on other essential activities.

The downside is our brain doesn't recognize good habits from bad. Our brain remembers the outcome of each habit, the **reward.** It retains the feedback. If it is positive, it acts automatically when the **cue** happens again. Thus, the habit forms and the neural pathway for the habit gets wired into our brain.

Habit formation requires a motivating component. As humans, we want positive reinforcement. When there is a lot of friction (i.e., when a task is difficult or makes us feel uncomfortable), we are less likely to do it. If we receive instant gratification from the behavior, we are more likely to continue the behavior.

I'm an emotional eater and I love food, especially sweets. Chocolate cake, snickerdoodle cookies, dark chocolate, and tiramisu are my jam. I've been known to eat when I'm stressed, bored, happy, or sad. If I have sweets in the house, I'll eat them.

My emotions trigger my behavior to eat sweets. Because I love the taste of sweets, I am instantly gratified, which encourages me to continue the behavior. Unfortunately, this gratification is fleeting, and I'm soon disgusted by my behavior. Sound familiar?

I've learned to keep sweets out of the house to avoid this type of behavior. They're a trigger. If I choose to have dessert, I will indulge outside the house and not bring it home. Likewise, if friends bring dessert when invited for dinner, I enjoy the dessert and send the rest home with them.

At the beginning of the chapter, I mentioned that environmental changes impact our behavior, impacting our habits. Old, less desirable habits can quickly replace positive habits. When you find yourself regressing into negative behavior patterns, try these tips:

ROUTINE, ROUTINE, ROUTINE

The sooner you can return to a familiar routine, the better. Creating a new routine, or re-establishing an old routine, will make it easier to regain momentum.

In the summer months, I walk my dog at 5:45 am, as the sun rises. Living in Texas, the temperature is tolerable in the early morning hours. By 8:00 am, the temp is close to 90 degrees with over 80 percent humidity.

This routine (habit) is easy to sustain through September before daylight savings time begins.

After the time change, when it's dark at 5:45 am, it's difficult to sustain my routine. So, I have to create a new habit. I may intend to walk later in the day, but without a specific routine, it's easy to get side-tracked. The day is over before I know it, and I haven't walked the dog.

My solution is to schedule a walk on my calendar. I've blocked the time, so I don't get side-tracked. An alarm on my phone is the **cue** to remind me to go for a walk. The **behavior** is the walk. The **reward** is the satisfaction that I've walked the dog.

Remember your habit's **Reward** is not the same as the Goal. For example, your new habit is to be more active (walk for 30 minutes every morning) with the goal of losing 50 pounds in six months. However, you will be overwhelmed if you focus on the big number without allowing yourself to enjoy your daily wins.

If your **goal** is to lose 50 pounds, and weight loss is slow, your perception is that it's taking forever to succeed. This can be frustrating and demotivating. Because we are motivated by instant gratification, a weight loss **reward** may not be realistic. Instead, consider focusing on how you feel when you're active. Think of the immediate benefits — you have more energy and flexibility, your clothes fit better, and you make better choices.

ESTABLISH A SLEEP SCHEDULE

When routines change, sleep schedules can change. If it's necessary to get up earlier in the morning to be active, adjust your bedtime routine accordingly. What time do you need to be in bed by to get seven to nine hours of rest? It may require beginning your nighttime regimen 30-45 minutes earlier. Set the alarm on your phone or smart watch to remind you of the new time. Since the days are longer in the summer, it may be dusk when you get to bed. If your bedroom is not dark enough, consider wearing a comfortable eye mask.

BE KIND TO YOURSELF

If you've had a setback due to a change in schedule or an indulgent vacation, give yourself some grace. Beating yourself up won't make you feel any better. Instead, if you're having difficulty getting back on track, reach out to a supportive friend or family member. It's never too late to reset. Start with your next meal.

Keep in mind that it takes time to develop new habits/routines. Everyone learns at different rates. Behavior is not changed overnight. Be patient with yourself. With repetition, your neural pathways will be strengthened, and the desired habit formation will occur.

Reflection questions:

1) What positive habits would you like to develop?

2) Identify the Cue, Behavior, and Reward of a current habit.

3) Identify each step (cue, behavior, reward) of the habits you wish to form.

_____

_____

_____

_____

_____

CHAPTER 5

ORGANIZE YOUR SUCCESS

How do you feel when you walk into an unorganized and cluttered room? I find it very stressful. If there are papers or clothes everywhere, it makes me anxious. I have difficulty focusing and am easily distracted.

How our spaces are arranged can impact our productivity which directly impacts our goal achievement. Think of how you respond when you walk into a messy room. Our actions are based upon our surroundings (cluttered or calm), how orderly or disorderly our spaces are, and the ease and the convenience of being in that space.

Set your environments up for success. Make it conducive to developing and maintaining healthy habits. Create spaces that are visually appealing and organized, so things are easy to find, rather than resembling a teenager's bedroom.

Here are some things to consider when setting yourself up for success:

START SMALL

If you have a lot to tackle, start with the area that is most aligned with your goals. For example, if you desire to lose weight, an organized kitchen is a good first place to start. Go through your refrigerator and discard expired condiments and tempting foods that do not align with your wellness goals.

Keep healthy options in clear containers, front and center (ex: cut up fruits and veggies) so that you see these treats when you open the fridge. Pre-cook and portion meal essentials (ex: rice or quinoa, oatmeal, chicken), and store in clear containers for easy meal preparation.

Once you've tackled the fridge, move to the pantry. Dispose of high-calorie temptations or put them in a less prominent location. Move healthier snacks to those eye-level shelves to encourage your good habits. Just as you did with the refrigerator, toss foods that are expired. Fill snack-size containers and bags with healthy snacks to prevent overeating and for easy grab and go as you are heading out the door.

> **How our spaces are arranged can impact our productivity which directly impacts our goal achievement.**

Next, organize drawers and cupboards to keep the kitchen tools and appliances that you use most often handy. Tools such as your favorite cutting boards, knives, peelers, measuring cups and spoons, a food scale, and appliances like an InstantPot, Slow Cooker, or Air Fryer.

ORGANIZED CLOSET

Having an organized closet will save you time getting ready in the morning and reduce stress. This is a task that might seem overwhelming, but if you start small, you'll be able to get it down more easily. Start with a section of the closet, such as a shelf, bar, or shoe cubby, and work through each section before moving to the next one. Donate or consign clothing that is the incorrect size, in good condition, outdated, or hasn't been worn in at least six months. These are clothes you're keeping for sentimental reasons (the prom dress or the slacks that fit you 10 years ago) or that you've forgotten about. Of course, keep your seasonal clothing.

ORGANIZE WORKSPACE

Whether you work from home or not, your work environment should be conducive to productivity. Keep items that you use often within reach and remember to put them back in the same spot when you're done with them. How many times has your phone wandered away from you? You don't want to dig through drawers or piles of paper to find what you need. Develop a simple system to organize your papers in files.

If most of your work is done on a computer, having your documents organized in folders is critical. If you're inundated with email, separate your messages into different folders (i.e., work, personal, etc.). Sifting through hundreds of messages to find what you're looking for is not only frustrating but unproductive. If you are self-employed, a virtual assistant can help you get and stay organized with just a few hours a month.

Natural lighting is best, but be sure to supplement it so that you can easily see what you are working on. You spend a considerable amount of time in your office and a comfy, ergonomic chair is essential to prevent joint, back, and neck pain.

Add some greenery to your workspace. Scientific research states that indoor plants relieve stress, increase productivity, reduce illness, create a more welcoming environment, clean the air, lower noise levels, and improve creativity. And it doesn't matter if it's an easy-care cactus or a temperamental orchid.

Keep something on your desk or on your wall that makes you smile and brings you joy. It could be a favorite inspirational quote, a picture of people or pets dear to you, or a small memento from a favorite trip.

Organizing your home and your workspace will bring you a sense of calm and order which will keep you focused on your goals.

Reflection
questions:

1) Which areas of your physical spaces might be limiting your success?

2) What steps can you take this week to make improvements?

3) Create an organization plan to tackle other areas.

CHAPTER 6

BE ACCOUNTABLE

Motivation is one of the most difficult emotions to maintain when you set a lofty goal. You may be all fired up when you start your journey, but you quickly lose your motivation and enthusiasm as time goes on.

Maybe your goal was to lose a substantial amount of weight, train for a marathon, or earn an incentive trip. What happened? If you're like many people, staying focused and motivated can be challenging, especially if you're relying on yourself for encouragement. When a bump in the road occurs, it can be difficult to get back on track and maintain a positive mindset. That's why accountability is so important for goal achievement.

When you're in the corporate world, your direct supervisor holds you accountable. If you're on a project team, your teammates hold you accountable. Knowing that someone has your back when things don't go as planned, problems arise, or mistakes happen, can mean the difference between success and failure. Without that support, it's possible that your business goals would not be met, and your performance would be negatively impacted.

Often when we set a personal goal, we don't think of having an accountability partner. We assume we have what it takes to get through tough situations. We may have the skills needed to navigate challenges, but our mindset is not in alignment.

For example, imagine that you've had a particularly stressful day at work. Instead of going for a walk when you get home, you kick off your shoes and open a bottle of wine. After the second glass you determine you're too tired to make dinner and decide to order a pizza. When the pizza arrives, you eat four pieces instead of the two you intended.

You turn on your favorite Netflix show and end up binge-watching several episodes until late in the evening. By the time you get to bed, it's hours past your normal bedtime. When the alarm goes off the next morning, you're exhausted and irritated with yourself for blowing it the previous evening. You tell yourself you have no willpower and that you'll never lose weight. When you get to work you discover a co-worker has brought donuts. Instead of refraining, you have two because you feel you are already so off track that it just doesn't matter.

Accountability partners can be close friends, family members, colleagues, advisors, and coaches. They may be going through or have been through a similar journey as you.

With an accountability partner, this situation would have a different outcome. For starters, a walking buddy would have encouraged you to join them on a walk. Then, if you had walked, your dopamine would have been higher, your stress relieved, and your decisions to stick with your healthy plan would have been easier to make. On those occasions when you do over-indulge, your accountability partner will be supportive and encouraging, to prevent you from further self-sabotage.

Accountability partners can be close friends, family members, colleagues, advisors, and coaches. They may be going through or have been through a similar journey as you. Regardless, they are someone you can trust to share your goals and hold you accountable. They will be your biggest cheerleader but will also expect you to do the work necessary to achieve your goals.

Communicating what you need from your accountability partner will set a clear expectation. Tell them you'd like a daily or weekly check-in with them to ensure you are staying on your path. Let them know you'll be honest about your efforts and will be grateful for their guidance. Your partner will appreciate your direction on how to work with you because then they know they are supporting you in the best way they can.

If you're struggling to achieve your goals, and lack motivation, it may be time to find an accountability partner. Think of the people in your life that are willing to encourage and support you to achieve your next goal.

Reflection questions:

1) List five people who would make a good accountability partner.

2) What do you need from your accountability partner?

3) When are you meeting with your accountability partner to get started on your goal?

SECTION II

Mindset

"Every day you have the power to choose."

Michelle Obama,
Former First Lady of the United States

CHAPTER 7

DEVELOP MINDFULNESS

Earlier, I touched upon the importance of mindfulness for creating sustainable goals. In this section, I'll take a deep dive into mindfulness and how it impacts all areas of life. Remember, our mindset determines the course of our life.

Mindfulness is the act of being aware and present in the current moment without judgment. When we are mindful and present, we can improve our overall health and wellness, relieve stress, improve sleep, and focus attention on what truly matters. Mindful individuals make healthier choices. They react more objectively to stress factors, choosing to focus on what they can control versus what they can't control.

Studies show that being present also makes us happier. When we're completely focused on what we're doing, we find more enjoyment in the activity. We're more inclined to do the activity and stick with it, even if it's a task we're not fond of.

For many individuals, exercise is not enjoyable. In the case of exercise, telling yourself that you hate exercise is not motivating. It's human nature to dislike activities that make us uncomfortable. We desire to do things that bring us joy and are comfortable.

What if the next time you are out for your daily walk you focused on your surroundings? Notice the colors, the sounds, and the smells, and really engage your senses. Would you feel differently about your walk? I venture to guess that you would. If anything, the walk would appear to go by more quickly.

Let's use housework as another example. Pushing a vacuum and dusting may be your least favorite activities. How would you feel if you focused on the progress of your cleaning instead of the actual cleaning process? Notice how the wood or glass starts to shine as you mop and dust. Notice how you feel when your environment is tidy. Are you more relaxed? How does the house smell? Does it smell fresh and clean? In my opinion, nothing smells better than a squeaky clean bathroom. Do I enjoy cleaning the bathroom? Not at all. However, I love the end result, the *"reward."*

Another benefit of being mindful and fully present is it forces us to slow down. In this busy world, we have a tendency to rush from one place to the next, often acting on auto-pilot. Our actions become so routine that we no longer pay attention to the process. Research shows that slowing down, being more present, and focusing on one task at a time, makes us more productive.

> **Mindfulness is the act of being aware and present in the current moment without judgment.**

This is a huge shift from 30+ years ago when employers considered multi-tasking a valuable skill. If you were skilled in multi-tasking you were considered more productive. I recently learned that multi-tasking was never supposed to be a skill for humans. IBM created the multi-tasking capability for computers because humans could not multi-task. How's that for a wake-up call! Instead of being more productive, multi-tasking creates inefficiency and stress.

When I was in my 20s, I prided myself on being an excellent multi-tasker. The more tasks I juggled at the same time, the better. Clearly, I was misguided in my belief. It is physically impossible to focus on two or more tasks at the same time. One task will hold your attention. When another task distracts you, your energy shifts to the other task. It's similar to being in two places at the same time. It's physically impossible.

If you find yourself stressed, lacking focus, making poor decisions, or not being productive, try these mindfulness techniques to become fully present:

BREATHE

Find a quiet, comfortable space to clear your mind. Focus on the breath. Take a deep breath in through your nose, and exhale slowly from your mouth. Notice how your diaphragm expands and contracts with each breath. If you find your mind wandering, gently redirect your focus to the breath. Continue for five minutes.

SENSE CONNECTION

Find a quiet, comfortable space to clear your mind. Notice your surroundings.

- Focus on five things you can see
- Focus on four things you can feel
- Focus on three things you can hear
- Focus on two things you can smell
- Focus on one thing you can taste

VISUALIZATION

Use your imagination for a brief escape. Find a comfortable space to relax. Close your eyes. Engage your senses. Now, imagine you're taking a walk, you pick a location. Focus on what you see, notice the light and how it illuminates your surroundings. Turn your attention to the sounds you would hear on your walk. Do you hear birds chirping, a stream skipping over the rocks, or an airplane flying overhead? Next, notice the scents around you — it may be a campfire, the salt of the ocean, or the aroma of a BBQ grill. How do you physically feel? Are you walking on a sidewalk, on a woodland path, or on a rocky beach? Can you feel the breeze on your face and the sun on your skin? Are you relaxed?

MUSIC

Listen to calming music. Gentle instrumental music of almost any genre is soothing and you can also find tonal music that is created to increase dopamine and serotonin levels to lift your mood.

GUIDED MEDITATION

Listen to a meditation app such as Calm, Headspace, Simple Habit, or Ten Percent Happier. Many health apps and coaches offer guided meditations online and you can listen anywhere.

PRACTICE YOGA

Yoga is not just for the physically fit. Everyone who has a yoga practice started with not knowing the forms and feeling unbalanced. Yoga classes are offered for all levels and are a great way to increase your awareness while creating stability and strength.

TAKE CONTROL

When you have an important task or project to complete, maintain your focus by eliminating distractions. Turn off your phone or put it in another room, silence notifications on your computer, or disconnect from all electronic devices entirely.

Mindfulness allows you to be fully present in your life. As you practice mindfulness you will find that you are more calm, able to accomplish your goals, and more aware of what is important to you. It is part of self-care.

Reflection questions:

1) What is one thing that you can commit to doing daily to be fully present?

2) How would practicing daily mindfulness impact your wellbeing, productivity, and relationships?

3) After one week of practicing mindfulness, list three situations where you chose to be mindful.

CHAPTER 8

BREAK YOUR BLOCKS

Have you ever taken the time to really think about why you do the things you do? Let me explain.

Back in the late 90s, I decided it was time to take back my health. My weight had gotten to an all-time high. I felt terrible. I was having stomach issues. My knees, back, and feet hurt. I was exhausted all the time. I started my weight loss journey with a friend. I lost 45 pounds and kept it off for three years.

In 2002 my husband and I moved from California to Texas. Neither of us had ever lived outside California. We took a leap of faith. If you've ever made a major move, you know, that everything changes. Not only does your environment change, but the culture and the way you live your life all change.

In California, I had been very active. I enjoyed long-distance bike riding, hiking, and walking. When we moved to Texas, all my habits changed. I continued with long-distance bike riding, but not as frequently. Hiking became a thing of the past. I walked when the weather permitted. Bottom line, I used the hot weather as an excuse to be less active.

I fell in love with Tex/Mex cuisine. Before I knew it, I had gained all my weight back plus 20 pounds. I felt miserable. I didn't take the time to ask myself why I was using food as a coping mechanism. Instead, I told myself I had no willpower.

Actually, if I had taken the time to really think about my behavior changes, I would have realized that I was stressed, homesick, and depressed. My new job was very stressful. I worked long hours. I missed the hills, mountains, ocean, and cooler weather of California. I greatly missed friends and family.

The truth was, I was depressed. Had I recognized the depression, and connected with a counselor or coach, I may have avoided a 65-pound weight gain and been a lot happier. I share this, not to say, shoulda, woulda, coulda, but to express how negative health behaviors stem from issues much deeper than a lack of willpower.

Fast forward to 2010; after seeing a picture of myself in a local newspaper article, I was horrified by my appearance. I barely recognized the person in the photograph. That was the wake-up call I needed. I started my weight loss journey for the second time. By the end of the year, I had lost 65 pounds. For the most part, I've kept it off.

The isolation during the COVID-19 Pandemic was a struggle. I gained 10 pounds during quarantine but have since lost that weight. Life is definitely a journey. Often the challenges we face, and the resulting behaviors, stem from something much bigger than what is presently occurring.

We don't recognize that we're blocked from achieving what we most desire by something other than a perceived lack of willpower. Maybe you've been a yo-yo dieter in the past. Maybe you struggle to reach that next business goal. You can see the desired result, but you just can't get there.

BUST A MYTH — IT TAKES WILLPOWER TO LOSE WEIGHT AND STAY ON A DIET

First, willpower is overrated. Individuals who appear to have a lot of willpower have the same willpower as individuals who seem to have none. Those with perceived willpower have learned to respond differently to outside influences and challenges. They have developed a positive, growth mindset. They are less likely to beat themselves up if they overindulge. They tend to bounce back more quickly after setbacks. Secondly, indefinitely staying on a diet is unrealistic for anyone. After all, the first three letters in the word diet are **die**. Diets are restrictive and unsustainable. The key to losing weight and keeping it off is developing sustainable lifestyle changes. Unless positive behavior change occurs, weight loss cannot be sustained.

THE #1 ROAD BLOCK

Fear. The word alone may make you uncomfortable. Fear is both a noun and a verb. As a noun, it is an unpleasant emotion caused by the belief that someone or something is dangerous and likely to cause pain or harm.

As a verb, fear is to be afraid of someone or something that can be potentially dangerous, painful, or threatening. Fear is the mind's way of keeping us safe. If we are in physical danger, it can be very effective.

The fight or flight response is triggered, causing adrenaline to rush through our bodies. This rush of adrenaline gives us quick energy to fight off or run away from captors. There is a downside to fear. It can prevent us from taking necessary action, keeping us stuck and preventing growth.

Would you be surprised to know that most individuals experience fear often? One of the most common fears is the fear of success. This may sound ridiculous. Who would be afraid of success? It's a misconception that everyone desires to be successful. While outwardly we all say we want to be successful, in actuality, our thoughts may include, *"What if I'm not ready for success? What if I can't handle success? What if success hurts my relationships? What if success forces me to do something I'm not comfortable with?"*

Fear of success can mask a fear of failure. Leaning into success may mean a discovery of incompetence. *"I'm not good enough. I'm not worthy of success."* These are lies we tell ourselves and that can be debilitating. We are good enough. We may not be highly skilled in everything we do, but we are worthy as human beings.

For most of my adult life, I've had a fear of success. I didn't realize it until I had a breakthrough during a coaching session during the pandemic. I had always considered myself a confident person. My belief, or so I thought, was if I put my mind to something, and gave 100 percent, I would be successful.

I felt this strongly when I was in my 20s. I was very confident regarding my job performance. Early in my retail career, my hard work was rewarded with multiple promotions. I was compensated well for my efforts. By the time I reached my 30s, my mindset began to shift. I had moved into a corporate role.

There I learned quickly that working hard was not enough; you had to play the game. I was never very good at corporate politics. I'm not a rule-breaker, but I'm also not a schmoozer. What you see is what you get. The toxic work environment began to erode my confidence in my abilities.

Externally I appeared to have it all together. To the outside world, I appeared very successful. I always felt I could do better. On the inside, I was stressed and anxious. When I left the corporate world in 2005 and migrated to direct sales, my confidence improved, but there was always an underlying fear that I would never be successful. As a result, I self-sabotaged my performance.

Fast forward to today. I am continuing to release the fear that I'm not good enough to be successful. I know this is a lie I tell myself. Some days are better than others. What I've learned is the importance of powering through the fear on the not-so-good days. It's okay to have fear. It's a human emotion. Don't let it debilitate you and prevent you from moving forward.

Fear is one of the largest roadblocks to being successful. Here are some additional scenarios of how fear can sabotage success.

- You were recently promoted and are fearful that you're not qualified for the job.

- You lost your job and are afraid that you'll never find another job.

- The thought of getting married makes you fearful. Your parents had a rocky marriage and eventually divorced. You don't want to follow in their footsteps.

- You desire to start your own business. You're afraid that your business will fail, that you'll lose your retirement savings, and let down your family.

Sometimes the fear of failure is masked by other challenges. Take weight gain for example. Consider you have a substantial amount of weight to lose but can't imagine reaching your goal. Your inner voice is telling you you're not good enough. As a result, fear causes you to self-sabotage with food.

Fear is one of the largest roadblocks to being successful.

Maybe you're struggling to get a promotion at work. You're fearful you're not good enough. As a result, you don't put yourself out there, staying under the radar. You use procrastination as an excuse. You tell yourself, *"I'm too busy to apply for that promotion. Now's not the right time."*

You may be drowning in debt. Your failure to adhere to a budget could also be a fear that you're not good enough. You spend money on things you can't afford, to temporarily make yourself feel better. Unfortunately, the feeling is short-lived and replaced with stress and desperation when you can't pay your bills.

Fear manifests in different ways. Common physical symptoms include anxiety, irritability, insomnia, migraines, and upset stomach, just to name a few. If this is relatable, it's time to seek help.

Chatting with a supportive friend or family member is a great place to start. A coach will recognize limiting beliefs that are preventing you from moving forward. Your health care provider can refer you to a counselor or therapist for chronic depression and anxiety.

Whether the desire is to get healthy, lose weight, achieve business goals, or improve relationships, a deep dive is needed to uncover your specific roadblocks. Once the roadblocks are removed, behavior change can begin. Through mindset shifts, goal setting, and accountability, sustainable healthy habits are created.

Reflection questions:

1) What has been your biggest challenge when it comes to goal achievement? Why?

2) What do you tell yourself to reinforce your fear or dispel it?

3) Name a time when you conquered a fear.

_____

_____

_____

_____

_____

CHAPTER 9

CUT UNHEALTHY TIES

Our past experiences shape our future. They create our perception of reality. Our parents, teachers, supervisors, partners, and friends impact how we see ourselves. If we felt safe, supported, and encouraged by our parents, we are more likely to have confidence as an adult.

A painful marriage or an unsupportive boss can create feelings of inadequacy and shame. A history of being abandoned, earlier in life, can lead to abandoning partners and friends or lashing out when feeling emotionally vulnerable. This can lead to a string of unhealthy relationships and self-sabotaging behavior.

Reflecting on past situations and viewing mistakes as learning experiences, can help us grow as individuals and establish boundaries within our lives. Unfortunately, for many, painful experiences from the past become a destination, and it becomes difficult to move forward in life. The need to relive the past becomes overwhelming. Emotions are triggered by sights, smells, and sounds. This can lead to chronic depression and Post-Traumatic-Stress-Disorder (PTSD).

There is also *"the grass is always greener"* mentality. Before I left the corporate world, my last position was in a very toxic environment. I dreaded going to work. I was completely burned out, working 80 hours/week. Everyone was stressed. Morale was at an all-time low. I would reminisce about my former job in California.

That job wasn't stressful. I had been in the position for several years and became very comfortable with my responsibilities, to the point of boredom. When I reminisced about that job, I focused on the positives and overlooked the factors that caused me to look for another position in the first place.

Sometimes, when we reminisce about the past, we can overlook the challenges and focus only on the good things that occurred. This is okay if we do it occasionally. When the reflection becomes a regular occurrence that only focuses on the positive, we create a false sense of reality.

According to psychcentral.com, here are some warning signs of living in the past:

- Your conversations revolve around a particular time, person, or situation.

- You are attracted to or attract, the same type of people that cause you pain.

- Your disagreements revolve around past arguments.

- You become easily bored or frustrated.

- You are constantly comparing your current situation to previous ones.

- Prior trauma or painful events replay in your mind.

- You create self-sabotaging behavior.

- Emotional triggers cause you to think about people or situations from the past.

- Relationships fill a void or prevent you from being alone with your thoughts.

- You are always "Waiting for the other shoe to drop" — expecting something bad to happen.

- You frequently feel anxious or act impulsively.

- You experience regret over impulsive choices.

- You have an "all or nothing" mindset about new people or new experiences.

- You prefer to avoid new people or new experiences.

If your past is preventing you from finding happiness and achieving success in your life, it's time to take action. You cannot change the past but you can impact the now and going forward.

A therapist, counselor, or coach can help identify experiences and triggers that are causing self-sabotaging behavior.

Setting boundaries of who you spend your time with provides an opportunity to heal.

Accepting the past is imperative. It can't be changed. Accepting that the past is over, allows time to grieve and release the pain.

Practicing mindfulness is about training the mind to stay in the present and remaining calm when experiencing emotional triggers. Mindfulness can be developed through meditation and visualization exercises. Refer to the techniques I discussed in Chapter 7.

Hit reset when challenges arise. *We are human and imperfect beings.* Let that sink in for a moment. You too are human! Be kind to yourself if you slip up, find yourself reliving the past, or reverting to old behavior patterns. Talk to yourself as you would a friend or family member you're close to.

> Reflecting on past situations and viewing mistakes as learning experiences can help us grow as individuals and establish boundaries within our lives.

Balance is key when working on self-improvement. It's okay to disconnect from social media, friends, or family to focus on self-care. When we are alone, we can get to know ourselves and give ourselves the attention and love we need to stop living in the past.

Reflection questions:

1) When do you reflect on the past?

2) How does reflecting on the past make you feel?

3) Do you find thoughts of the past encroaching on how you view the future?

_____

_____

_____

_____

CHAPTER 10

SPEAK KINDLY TO YOURSELF

With so much unrest in the world, it's easy to jump on the negativity bandwagon. When we're tired, stressed, or even bored, these negative feelings can compound, and the things we say to ourselves are often untrue and unkind.

When you are feeling vulnerable, give yourself some grace. These negative thoughts can become a self-fulfilling prophecy. Often, they are so ingrained in our subconscious that we don't easily recognize them. When we practice mindfulness, we create awareness of negative thoughts and behavior patterns. It's human nature to become your worst critic, but instead, be kind to yourself. Once we recognize these unhelpful thoughts we can ask ourselves if what we're saying is really true or just a lie we're telling ourselves. We can flip our negative thoughts by adding "yet" to the end of each statement.

"I have no willpower, yet."

"I can never lose weight, yet."

"I haven't been successful, yet."

"I've never had enough money, yet."

Flipping our thoughts takes practice. The good news, with repetition, we can change our mindset and build confidence.

We tend to treat ourselves far worse than we do others. We set unrealistic expectations of ourselves. When we fail to meet these expectations, we feel like a failure. Over time, this type of behavior can impact our confidence, self-worth, and ultimately, our actions. What we think about impacts our belief system which drives our behavior. Imagine if a family member or close friend treated themselves the way you treated yourself? What would you say to them? Would you be judgmental or would you be supportive and encouraging?

When situations do not go as planned, instead of beating yourself up, ask yourself, "What did I learn from this experience? How can I make a difference next time?" Be curious and not judgmental. This takes practice but is doable. The more you do it, the easier it becomes.

Letting go of the negative and focusing on the positive promotes growth and a healthy mindset. In the next chapter, I'll discuss how external stimulants, such as the news, social media, and other people's opinions and expectations can hinder our mindset and positive growth. You'll build your confidence and your success rate by learning to flip your negative thoughts to create an empowering mindset.

THE POSITIVITY RIPPLE

Have you ever been around someone that has a cool vibe? Let's call her Jane. Jane is happy. She's a glass-half-full gal, radiating positivity. Others are drawn to her. She has a unique sense of style and is not concerned about what others think of her. Jane projects confidence but is not cocky. You want to be around Jane. She makes you feel good. Her positive energy is contagious.

Now imagine a very different type of person. Let's call her Cathy. Drama follows her wherever she goes. It's like a cloud. There's always a problem. She views the world negatively. We're all doomed. Others are out to get her. Cathy attracts similar-minded people into her sphere of influence, the Negative Naysayers. Misery loves company. If you're like Jane, the Cathys of the world can suck the life out of you.

So, let me ask you, how do you show up in the world? You may feel that on some days you have a little Jane in you. On other days you may be more like Cathy. That's normal. We all have good days and bad days. My objective is to make you aware of how your energy is influencing your mindset and actions.

You may have heard of the Law of Attraction. By definition, the Law of Attraction is based on the belief that positive or negative thoughts bring positive or negative experiences into a person's life. The belief is based on the principle that people and their thoughts are made of "pure energy."

Through the process of like energy attracting like energy, a person can influence their life by their thoughts, what they say, and their actions. For

> **What we think about impacts our belief system which drives our behavior.**

example, if a person is positive, looks at challenges as learning experiences, and believes they can have great health, wealth, and positive relationships, they will attract the things they desire. Techniques such as positive affirmations and "I AM" statements help frame the mindset to attract their desires.

In Hinduism and Buddhism, a similar concept of the Law of Attraction is expressed by karma. Karma is the sum of a person's actions in this and previous states of existence, viewed as deciding their fate in future existences. You've heard the phrase, what goes around comes around. If you're negative and treat people poorly, others will reciprocate this same behavior towards you.

For many, there is the belief in destiny or fate. Our destiny or fate is predetermined. Our actions lead us to that fate. We may have some impact on the steps we take to reach our destiny, but we cannot impact our fate.

In terms of behavioral science, what we think about impacts our belief system which drives our behavior. For example, if we tell ourselves repeatedly that we can never be truly happy or successful, these thoughts will become our belief system. This belief system will subconsciously sabotage our behavior, so happiness and success will elude us.

Now that you are aware there are forces that impact our beliefs and behavior, how do you choose to show up in the world? Will you be a Jane or a Cathy? Are you happy with the direction of your life? Are you surrounded by Janes or Cathys?

AFFIRMATIONS

When you are in your happy and contented "Jane" mode it is easy to think positive thoughts that spur you on to achieve your goals. But, when challenges arise, it can be difficult to think positively, especially when we do not feel that we're capable of achieving our goals and desires.

One way to shift our negative mindset to a positive mindset is through affirmations. Affirmations are carefully formatted statements, repeated frequently, that are written down and stated in the present tense as if they are occurring now. They are always positive, personal, and specific.

An example is, *"I am at my healthy weight and feel fantastic! I have abundant energy and feel confident."* What makes affirmations work is repetition and linking the affirmation to an emotion. Think of it as creating a habit for your brain. By repeating a positive affirmation frequently, you are creating and strengthening a neural pathway in your brain. Attaching emotion to the affirmation makes it easier to visualize.

With enough repetition, this thought process will become automatic. Your brain will react as if you've already accomplished what you set out to do. Your actions will reflect a positive mindset. In this example, you'll make healthier choices. These choices will help you reach your goal weight.

For more information about positive affirmations, check out the following articles:

https://blog.mindvalley.com/positive-affirmations/

https://www.huffpost.com/entry/affirmations_b_3527028

You can create your own affirmations. They can be as simple as "I am a healthy person who loves fruit and vegetables," which will help steer you away from cookies and candy. If you are striving to be more fiscally responsible you can state, "I spend my money wisely and love watching my savings grow."

Each morning, as I eat my breakfast, I spend time in devotional study and repeating affirmations. My affirmations apply to all areas of my life. They keep me focused on my vision and goals. When I was in the direct sales industry, I earned many incentive trips for my performance. Affirmations were instrumental to my success, by keeping me focused on my goals. How could affirmations help you achieve your goals?

Reflection questions:

1. Take a moment and think of how you speak to yourself when things go wrong?

2. Would you speak that way to a loved one or a colleague?

3. Create an affirmation that you can use to start your day.

CHAPTER 11

CONTROL THE NOISE

Do you ever feel like your brain is so full of junk that you can't focus? You have so many thoughts swirling around in your head. There's an ongoing checklist in your brain, maybe on paper too, that is never completed. You always have something to do. It's exhausting and stressful.

I've had to learn how to manage my thoughts in order to remain positive, productive, and stress-free. I have a tendency to set very high expectations for myself. It's one thing to hold yourself to a high standard. It's another to hold yourself to an unrealistic expectation of performance. This is a form of perfectionism, which is actually a fear of rejection.

During a conversation with my coach, I discovered that my tendency to set ridiculously high expectations of myself is a way of getting attention. This is a by-product of my relationship with my mother. She suffered from mental illness. I would describe my mother's personality as one of two extremes. She was either: incredibly happy, supportive, and loving, or she would shut me out completely.

I remember a time when I was in Junior High School when she didn't speak to me for a week. I had done something to upset her. I think I forgot my parent's anniversary. She reacted by treating me as if I didn't exist. Growing up, this was very confusing and upsetting. When she was in a mood, I would try to engage her in conversation but would be ignored. In hindsight, I can see she was going through a difficult time and could not process her emotions in a healthy way. This behavior created a need in me to be noticed.

What's interesting is I never realized this need manifested into unrealistic expectations of myself. This fear of rejection was so deeply buried that it took my coach to recognize the signs. As this situation illustrates, deeply rooted fears are often masked by layers of varying behavior. The noise in my head was telling me I had to accomplish an unrealistic amount of tasks. This noise was a reaction to a deeply buried fear of rejection.

Mental to-do lists are not the only form of noise. The news, social media, as well as other people's opinions and expectations all, generate noise. With the invention of cell phones, instant messaging, and FaceTime, we have become too accessible. Unless we set healthy boundaries, others have access to us 24/7. Those closest to us offer opinions that generate stress. This is exacerbated by the news and social media, creating a toxic overload.

When I find my brain full of noise, including an unrealistic checklist of expectations, I recognize it's time to reset. If this resonates with you, here are some tips for letting go of noise:

1) Take a moment to do some deep breathing. This will lower your blood pressure and help you to relax.

2) If you're spiritual, pray. The act of letting go and surrendering toxic emotions to a higher being is freeing and comforting.

3) Listen to soothing music. This can help quiet the brain.

4) Take a warm bath or shower.

5) Do a quick brain dump. Grab a piece of paper and write down all the thoughts that are swirling in your head. They don't have to make sense. Jot them down anyway.

6) Go outside. Natural light is a mood elevator.

7) Go for a walk. Focus on nature. What do you hear? What do you smell? What do you see?

8) Call a supportive friend.

9) Drink a cup of decaf tea.

10) Close your eyes and visualize that you're in your happy place. What does it look like? Notice your surroundings. Is it nature, people, or buildings you see? What do you feel? Is there a warm breeze caressing your skin? Do you hear birds chirping, waves crashing, etc.? What do you smell? Spend a couple of minutes in your happy place and then slowly open your eyes.

Things to avoid or limit access to:

1) Television and social media — Both can over stimulate the brain.

2) Caffeine — Caffeine is a stimulant. If you're overstimulated, this will increase anxiety.

3) Processed sugar — Avoid sugary foods and beverages. Processed sugar is a stimulant. It may increase your energy temporarily but will act as a depressant when the effects wear off.

4) Alcohol — Alcohol is a depressant. It may relax you temporarily but will increase your anxiety in the long run. It can also prevent you from getting a good night's rest.

Taking time to breathe and relax is a form of self-care. It is essential to overall health and well-being. When we take time to care for ourselves, reducing the noise, we can better care for others and be the best version of ourselves.

> **The news, social media, as well as other people's opinions and expectations all, generate noise.**

Over the past couple of years, I've made significant improvement in letting go of things outside of my control. When I feel myself getting anxious, I make a list of things within my control and a list of things outside my control. I focus on those things I can impact, how I respond to situations and my choices. I let go of everything else.

Sometimes there are a lot of prayers involved, as it's not always easy. However, the more you practice this, the more equipped you become in handling the unexpected. Are you spending too much time and energy on things outside of your control? Are you anxious, stressed, depressed, or frustrated? Do you find it difficult to focus on the positive? If the answer is yes, it's time to let go and focus on what you can control.

Here are some tips for letting go.

1) Focus on the positive. Start by practicing gratitude. What is one thing you're thankful for? Keep a gratitude journal by your bed.

2) Practice mindfulness. Become aware of where you are and what you're doing, without becoming overly reactive or overwhelmed by what's going on around you. Be present. Approach your observations with curiosity, not judgment.

3) Visualize the desired outcome. Let go of what could go wrong.

4) Set boundaries. Be intentional about how you spend your time and who you spend it with.

5) Create a fear list. What are you most fearful of? Writing down fears brings them to light. Most often fears are unrealistic.

6) Get support. If letting go is a struggle, reach out to a close friend, family member, pastor, or coach.

Remember, you will have good days and challenging days. Appreciate that you're a work in progress. Don't pass judgment on yourself. Embrace where you are. After all, you're human.

Reflection questions:

1) What creates stress in your life?

2) What is one small action you can take this week to manage stress?

_____

_____

_____

_____

_____

CHAPTER 12

SET PRIORITIES & CREATE BOUNDARIES

Are you stressed, overcommitted, burned out, and exhausted? If you're like many business owners and executives, you feel like a hamster on the wheel, constantly going, going, and going but never getting anywhere. This is your reality, most days, if not every day. This is a classic sign of life being out of balance.

When our lives are out of balance, there are typically one or two areas that are monopolizing our time. If not adjusted, this lifestyle can lead to serious physical and emotional health problems, as well as relationship and productivity challenges.

Finding balance is about setting priorities. When I was in the corporate world, I allowed my job to take precedence over everything in my life. I was always working or thinking about work. I had very little energy left for my husband. As a result, my health and marriage suffered. Setting priorities creates the precedence of what is most important at a given time. It is a form of boundaries.

For many individuals, being likable, helpful, and supportive, are qualities that are important. When we say yes, it is often with these attributes in mind. Saying yes can be very rewarding when we feel needed and appreciated. It can also be a source of stress if we are feeling overwhelmed and overscheduled. Stress is one of the greatest inhibitors to joy and happiness.

There are exceptions. Healthy stress, when working toward a deadline, can be a great motivator. When stress begins to impact our well-being and relationships, it's time to set boundaries.

Saying no is one of the best boundaries you can set for yourself. We often think, that saying no means we're a bad person. We're not being helpful. We may even think we're being selfish. Saying no is not selfish. It's saying that we're putting ourselves first and we value our time. When we set healthy boundaries, we are not only taking care of ourselves, but we're better able to take care of those most important to us.

When we say yes to something, we're saying no to something else. By always saying yes, we're allowing others to control our lives. If we feel there is not enough time in the day for what is important, that is on us. We control our schedule. It is our choice how we spend our time.

> **Saying no is one of the best boundaries you can set for yourself.**

A big Ah-Ha for me, was when I realized that setting boundaries earned me respect instead of resentment. One of my biggest takeaways from the pandemic was the need to have downtime. As a hyper-achiever and an extrovert, I gain energy from people and being busy.

This is the complete opposite of my husband, who is an introvert. He needs downtime, away from others, to rest and recharge. Being around a lot of people and having a very full schedule depletes his energy. During the lockdown, when I was forced to slow down, I began to recognize how much I enjoyed the time to relax and practice self-care. Self-care for me includes puzzling, reading, and going for long walks. When I had time to do these things, I was much happier.

When the world reopened, I found my schedule becoming very full again. I recognized how much I missed these simple pleasures. I now make it a practice to not overschedule myself on nights and weekends. I schedule time for self-care. I've jokingly told my husband that I'm becoming more of an introvert.

If I find my schedule becoming too full, I politely decline invitations. When I am transparent about my reasons, I generate respect. Others appreciate my honesty. I am not criticized for saying no. As a result, I've let go of my fear of being judged by others for saying no.

Do you have a fear of saying no? If so, it's time to let it go and set boundaries to create balance in your life. No one cares that you say no. They're more concerned with their actions. If you don't believe me, that's fear telling you otherwise. Here are some tips for establishing balance:

1) Create a schedule

Take a piece of paper and divide it into three columns.

    a. Left column   High priority tasks (ex: work, kid activities, doctor's appointments, self-care, grocery shopping, etc.). Yes, I did include self-care. It's mandatory!

    b. Middle column   Medium priority tasks that need to be accomplished in the next few weeks but are not urgent.

    c. Right column   Include all low priority tasks (ex: clean out the closet, organize spice drawer, etc.).

On the backside of your paper, jot down all the repetitive tasks that occupy your day. Include getting ready for work and all the time suckers, such as social media, email, TV, and computer games.

Once you've created your lists, place your High, Medium, and Low priority tasks on a month at-a-glance calendar. It will provide an excellent visual of available time blocks. If you have limited or no availability, it's necessary to assess how much time you're spending on time suckers. You may be surprised at how many hours you are spending, scrolling social media and watching Netflix.

2) If you regularly have back-to-back meetings throughout the day, schedule 20-30 minute breaks between meetings to run to

the restroom, grab a snack, refill water, stretch your legs, and check your email. If you're thinking 10-15 minutes will suffice, consider what will happen when a meeting runs long. No breaks!

3) Be sure to set office hours. If you don't, you're telling your co-workers and your clients that you're available anytime.

4) Set clear boundaries. Stop being a people pleaser.

5) Let go of what you can't control. You are not responsible for the whole world, just your little piece of it.

As a friend said, "No is a complete sentence." Use that magic word to help you set and maintain your boundaries for a balanced life.

Reflection
questions:

1) Think of something you said "Yes" to but really didn't want to.

2) Think of how you could say "No" to that same situation.

3) List one example of when you thoughtfully said "No" to a request for your time, talent, or treasure.

4) After you said no, how did you feel in the moment? How did you feel a few days later?

_____

_____

_____

_____

_____

CHAPTER 13

NEVER GIVE UP!

Life can be overwhelming. At times, it may feel as if nothing is going right, remaining positive seems impossible, and everything seems hopeless. I've been there, and it's not a fun place to be. In fact, it sucks. If you're there right now, I feel your pain. It's absolutely real, and no one can truly relate unless they've been there. Here's my story…

On New Year's Eve 2020, I had a total knee replacement. If you've had a joint replaced you know that the post-surgery pain is very intense. Fortunately, there are strong narcotics that help with the discomfort.

However, I am allergic to most narcotics, and I had a severe allergic reaction to the narcotic that I was taking in the hospital. As a result, I was without pain meds for eight hours post-surgery, before a substitute medication that I could tolerate was approved.

Since my pain could not be managed, what should have been a one-night hospital stay turned into three nights. I am not a crier. In fact, I've been told I'm very strong and stoic. Well, I'm here to tell you, I was a blubbering mess. I was screaming and sobbing. I literally went crazy. I scared the nurses. I can only imagine what the other patients thought.

This was not my finest hour. I believe it was the lowest point in my life. I kept telling myself I was crazy to have had my knee replaced. I couldn't see past the pain. I could think of nothing positive. When it was apparent that my stay would be prolonged, the medical team was concerned that I was not moving my joint.

By the third day the hospital doctor informed me that if I did not get up and walk down the hall, I would be sent to a rehab facility for a week. That was the wake-up call I needed. I refused to go to a rehab facility. I just wanted to go home. The mind is a powerful thing; on the morning of the 4th day I told myself I was getting up, no matter what. I did. Not only did I make it to the bathroom, but I also walked down the hall. The nurses and doctor were amazed.

Fast forward to home. It was the first visit from my in-home physical therapist. My range of motion was significantly below where it should be. My pain level, although improved, was not fully managed. Although I could walk better with a walker, my range of motion was still well below where it should have been. The therapist expressed concern that I might have to have my knee surgically bent if I could not improve my range of motion.

> When going through times of extreme stress, it's important to focus on what we have as opposed to what we're lacking.

Thoughts of excruciating pain and an additional six-week delay in my recovery sent me into a panic. I went to that dark place again. I failed to see the progress I was making in my overall strength and movement. All I could think about was the fact that I couldn't get my range of motion to where it needed to be. I felt like a loser. Why could other people do this, and I couldn't?

It took a good friend of mine to give me another wake-up call. She reminded me that I had gotten through other difficult times in the past because of my strong faith. She reminded me that God was with me and would get me through this. I needed to stop fighting and let Him handle this. HELLO! Get over yourself and give it to God.

We all go through tough times. Whatever is going on in your life, please know this, you **WILL** get through it! Sometimes it takes the lowest point in your life to make you appreciate what you have and realize that you can overcome anything if you put your mind to it.

I do believe that once I got out of my own miserable head and let God handle the situation, I was able to improve and move on. You may not have a similar belief system. That's okay. Whatever you believe in, you can overcome anything if you put your mind to it. Negativity breeds negativity. Finding one small thing to be thankful for can start to move the barometer.

When going through times of extreme stress, it's important to focus on what we have as opposed to what we're lacking. By doing so, we can increase our happiness by 25 percent, according to University of California Psychology Professor, Dr. Robert Emmons.

In his book, *Thanks!: How Practicing Gratitude Can Make You Happier*, Dr. Emmons states that a person who experiences gratitude handles everyday stress more effectively, can show increased resilience in trauma-induced stress, and is more likely to have better physical health, including recovering more quickly from illness.

If you're struggling to find something to be thankful for, remember this…you're alive! That counts for something. You have a roof over your head. You have clean drinking water. You have clothes on your back. You have food. Sometimes it takes the most basic things we take for granted, to make us realize that we have many things to be thankful for.

Once we start focusing on these things, it becomes easier to find other simple things to be grateful for: a steaming cup of coffee, a hot shower, or a beautiful sunrise after a week of rain. The amazing thing about our brains is that we can retrain them quickly. When we repeat the same behavior consistently, we create strong neural pathways that focus on the new behavior.

Challenges are a part of life. How we react to challenges can set us up for success or failure. The first step to overcoming challenges is to determine if the obstacle is within our control. If it is, how can we positively impact the roadblock? Having a positive mindset can shift our thinking from something negative to a learning experience. If the obstacle is outside our control, let it go. It's not worth the energy.

Whatever you do, never give up! You are stronger than you know. If no one's told you lately, you are amazing. You've got this!

Reflection questions:

1) If a loved one were struggling with a significant challenge, how would you encourage them?

2) How can you use this same behavior for yourself?

3) Record your "Gratitude" each night before you go to sleep. Write down the big and small things that had a positive impact on your day.

_____

_____

_____

_____

_____

SECTION III

Emotional Self-Care

"I don't have to chase extraordinary moments to find happiness — it's right in front of me if I'm paying attention and practicing gratitude."

Brené Brown, Inspirational Author

CHAPTER 14

GO ON VACATION

We live in a stressful world. Individuals and technology are constantly vying for our attention. We've become so accessible that it's difficult to unplug. If you're an entrepreneur, small business owner, or in the corporate sector, you may feel that you're always working.

Finding a work-life balance can be challenging. As mentioned earlier, If boundaries are not set and balance is not maintained, it can lead to serious mental and physical health problems.

I subscribe to Marie Forleo's newsletter. She is the host of MarieTV, an entrepreneur, philanthropist, and *New York Times* best-selling author of the book, *Everything is Figureoutable*. In one of her newsletters, she described how it felt to be on her annual company summer break, with no meetings and no email:

"That first year, it was SCARY to shut down for a full two weeks. I had the same feelings as you:

> **Guilt** *over taking time off and not being available 24/7*
> **Fear** *that I'd miss an opportunity or let down a client*
> **Stress** *about having to "make up for lost time" later*
> **Self-doubt** *that taking time off meant I was lazy or uncommitted*

But here's the thing...

If we want anything to change — within our lives, our businesses, or our society — we have to take action and lead the way."

This really resonated with me because it is easy for me to work all the time as I'm a solopreneur with a strong work ethic. My careers in corporate retailing and direct selling created the mindset that if I'm not doing an income-producing activity, I'm not making money. While this may be true, there's WAY more to life than just work.

If you're reading this and are experiencing the same feelings as Marie describes, it's time to go on vacation! You may be telling yourself, *"I don't have time for a vacation. Now is not the right time. I'll go on vacation once I accomplish XYZ."*

The problem with this mindset is there's never a right time. You'll always have things to do. If you put off vacation due to a particular project, you may complete the project but something else will come up to monopolize your time.

I admit, that I often have this mindset before I go on vacation. I stress about getting everything wrapped up ahead of time. What I've found is when I've felt the most stressed out, that is exactly when I need to take a break.

Vacation is important for many reasons...

1) Vacation makes people happier. Happier people tend to be healthier and lead more productive lives.

2) Vacation reduces stress. Stress, if not properly managed, can lead to heart disease, diabetes, obesity, certain types of cancer, and emotional problems. Therefore, vacation can improve your health.

3) Vacation provides you with an opportunity to connect with family and friends.

4) Vacation provides the opportunity to travel to destinations you've never been before.

5) Studies show that vacation time can actually improve your productivity, by allowing you to recharge and refocus.

6) Vacation improves mindset by providing an opportunity to relax and let go of negative stress factors. When we're on vacation, we're more inclined to be fully present. It's easier to let go of what we can't control. When we're rested, we make better choices and are happier.

If boundaries are not set and balance is not maintained, it can lead to serious mental and physical health problems.

You can get the same benefits from a staycation or a destination-cation. The key is to fully disconnect. If it's been a while since you've taken time off, it may be time to plan your next vacation. You'll be glad you did!

Reflection
questions:

1) How often do you schedule downtime to refresh and recharge?

2) What vacation will you take this year?

3) Imagine your perfect vacation, free from digital distraction. Where would it be, who would be with you, and what would you be doing?

_____

_____

_____

_____

_____

CHAPTER 15

LAUGH OUT LOUD

Whenー was the last time you had a good belly laugh? Not a chuckle, but the laughter that made it difficult to breathe, your stomach and face hurt, and you were crying. There may have been some snorts in there for good measure.

When I was healing from my knee replacement, laughter was integral in raising my spirits. There wasn't much to laugh about in my recovery. However, I found solace in binge-watching episodes of *Schitt's Creek*. For hours, I would take my mind off the pain and frustration by laughing with the Rose family. It definitely was my therapy, helping me get through a very dark period.

You may have heard that laughter is the best medicine. Studies show that laughter truly is good for your health. According to HelpGuide.org, there are many physical health benefits to laughter.

1) Laughter relaxes the entire body, releasing stress and anxiety. In fact, a good laugh can keep your muscles relaxed for up to 45 minutes after.

2) Laughter boosts the immune system by decreasing stress hormones and increasing immune cells and infection-fighting antibodies.

3) Laughter releases endorphins, the body's natural, feel-good chemicals. Endorphins create an overall sense of well-being and have been known to temporarily relieve pain.

4) Laughter protects the heart by improving the function of blood vessels and increasing blood flow which can help protect against heart attack and other cardiovascular problems.

5) Laughter burns calories. One study found that laughing for 10 to 15 minutes per day can burn approximately 40 calories. This could be enough to lose three to four pounds over a year's time. This should not give you an excuse to ditch your gym membership!

6) Laughter is one of the quickest ways to diffuse anger. It helps to put problems into perspective and reduce confrontations without holding onto bitterness and resentment.

Studies show that laughter truly is good for your health.

7) Laughter may help you live longer. A study in Norway showed that people with a sense of humor outlived those who did not laugh often. This is especially true for individuals battling cancer.

In addition to physical health benefits, laughter has many mental health benefits.
1) Laughter adds joy to life.
2) Laughter has been proven to reduce anxiety and tension.
3) Laughter relieves stress.
4) Laughter is a mood elevator.
5) Laughter strengthens resilience.

The next time you're stressed, frustrated, or on your last nerve, consider watching your favorite comedy, listening to your favorite comedian, or reaching out to a friend with a sense of humor. Not only will you relieve your stress and frustration, but you will impact your overall health and wellness.

Reflection questions:

1) What's your type of humor?

2) How will you make yourself laugh this week?

3) Who do you love to laugh with?

CHAPTER 16

10 WAYS TO EXPERIENCE JOY

Joy, by definition, is a feeling of great pleasure and happiness. From a spiritual perspective, it is a good feeling in your soul. Joy is long-lasting and warms the heart.

When experiencing joy, you may also experience happiness. However, this is not always the case. You may have internal peace about a situation but may not be happy. From a biblical perspective, the prophet Paul felt joy while he was in prison. He was not happy to be in prison, but he was at peace and joyful knowing that he would be free from suffering one day, having been saved through Christ Jesus.

You may not be entirely happy with your current situation. However, you may feel a sense of peace and joy, knowing that your current situation is preparing you for something better.

Because happiness can be fleeting, striving to live a joyful life can provide peace and contentment during life's challenges. Here are some ways to create joy in your life:

1. Buy experiences, not possessions. The anticipation of an experience can be as valuable a source of happiness as the experience itself. Memories of the experience can bring lasting joy.

2. Focus on what you're good at. Spend your energy on things that are your strengths. When you focus on your strengths, you experience less depression and create satisfaction which leads to joy.

3. *Never* sacrifice *"Me Time."* Prioritize what brings you joy. Schedule it. You're worth it!

4. Rise above the difficult situation. Negative experiences can help us grow and learn. Instead of focusing on the *"shoulda, coulda, woulda,"* focus on what you've learned. You can't change the past. You can impact the future.

> **Because happiness can be fleeting, striving to live a joyful life can provide peace and contentment during life's challenges.**

5. Contribute your time and talents. Studies show that doing things for other people you know makes you feel the happiest and most joyful. This is not at the expense of *"Me Time."*

6. Focus on your relationships with your spouse, family, and friends. Studies show that relationships with those you spend the most time with will decline in quality over time. View these relationships as an objective third party. Consider how you can improve your connection with your loved ones rather than just maintaining it on auto-pilot.

7. Make eye contact, smile, and be kind to the people you encounter daily. Your awareness will spark joy for them and you.

8. Bring joy to your everyday tasks by listening to music or a favorite podcast while commuting to work, cooking dinner, or doing other household chores.

9. Smile anyway. Smiling can reduce your heart rate during stressful moments.

10. Laugh. As mentioned previously, laughter really is the best medicine.

Reflection
questions:

1) What is something that brings you joy?

2) How will you experience joy this week?

3) How will you share joy with someone else this week?

CHAPTER 17

INVEST IN YOURSELF

In July of 2021, I did something I'd never done before. I took a risk and made a sizable investment in myself and my business. I invested in a three-month intensive personal development and coaching program. I'd been contemplating the investment for months.

Although I had a strong desire to join the program, I was afraid of what it could mean for me personally as well as for my business. Yes, the price tag made me GULP, but what I discovered was it wasn't really about the money. It was about the fear of failure. Crazy as it sounds, my fears revolved around what I would discover about myself and how I would show up in my business.

As discussed earlier, fear of failure impacts many individuals. For some, it's the fear of success. These fears can lead to inaction and the inability to achieve desired goals. Common negative thought patterns include: *"I'm not ready. I don't have the money. I don't have the skills or knowledge needed to be successful. Now is not the right time."*

These thoughts are not facts. We tell ourselves these untruths to keep ourselves comfortable and safe. Putting ourselves out there, being vulnerable, and taking risks is scary.

The key to overcoming fear is to recognize that it exists. For many of us, these underlying fears are buried under a mountain of unhealthy behavior, including negative thought patterns. By talking to a trusted friend, family member, pastor, coach, or therapist you can help uncover the underlying issue.

When have you invested in yourself? Investing in yourself means doing anything that contributes to your long-term well-being. This takes commitment and courage. It doesn't necessarily mean investing thousands of dollars or focusing on material things. It's about investing in your overall health and wellness, both mentally and physically.

> **Investing in yourself means doing anything that contributes to your long-term well-being.**

Think about what inspires you and brings you joy. Identify the skills or education that could help you achieve your goals and dreams. Consider how you can become your best self and show up in the world as the unique, amazing individual that you are.

By investing in yourself, you can be a better human, parent, sibling, spouse, friend, co-worker, business executive, or entrepreneur. You can more effectively serve others and your community.

You can invest in yourself in different ways.

1) Read self-improvement books. We can always learn and grow. What is something that is challenging for you? Read about it!

2) Take a course at a local college or community center. Learn a new skill or improve on an existing one.

3) Develop an appreciation for the arts. Tour a museum, take a painting or sculpting class or go to the symphony or local theater.

4) Focus on your health and wellness. If this is a challenge, hire a coach, get an accountability partner, join a gym, or take a

fitness class. Get your ZZZs. A good night's rest helps repair your body, brings mental clarity, contributes to maintaining a healthy immune system, and improves your mindset, which guides you to make better choices.

5) Schedule time to relax. Do something just for you...take a bubble bath, go for a walk, get a mani-pedi, listen to your favorite music, meditate, pray, or read a book.

6) Set healthy boundaries. Learn to say no. Being over-scheduled is not only stressful but can prevent you from taking time for yourself. If this is a struggle, check out Dr. Henry Cloud's book, *Boundaries*.

7) Spend time with others who motivate and inspire you to be your best self.

Investing in you is not selfish, it is necessary. Whether it is taking the time for your morning meditation or signing up for a language course, by investing in yourself, you are becoming more valuable to everyone around you.

Reflection
questions:

1) What do you do daily that is just for you?

2) When and what was your most recent self-investment?

3) How will you invest in yourself this week?

_____

_____

_____

_____

CHAPTER 18

CREATE SUSTAINABLE HAPPINESS

You may have heard the saying, "Happiness is an inside job." This implies that we create our own happiness, or it's something we are born with. Here are some statistics...

1) Approximately 50 percent of the variation in happiness levels among individuals, is a direct result of genetics. Yes, the happiness gene does exist, and some lucky individuals are blessed with it.

2) Life circumstances account for approximately 10 percent of the variation in happiness levels.

3) The remaining 40 percent is up to us, meaning, we have control over our happiness.

The biggest contradiction to these statistics is corporate marketing campaigns that claim their products generate happiness. For example, unwinding at the end of a long day in our comfy rope chair hammock will bring a smile to your face, or, our fun, breezy print sheets will instantly lighten your mood. I don't know about you, but if I've had one of those days, looking at bed sheets in a breezy print (what the heck is a breezy print anyway?) isn't going to make me feel light-hearted and care-free.

When I was in a toxic corporate environment, I was particularly irritated by individuals with a sunny disposition. You know who I mean, that annoying Suzy Sunshine. She's always smiling and happy. Life is fantastic! She never has an unkind word to say about anyone. How can she be so happy all the time? I mean, REALLY! It's so annoying. She's such a people pleaser, just trying to be the center of attention and get ahead. What a brown noser!

When you're in a toxic work environment, surrounded by negative people, it's easy to become negative, especially when you're stressed and burned out. You have little tolerance for Suzy Sunshine. The sad reality is, that if I had spent more time with Suzy and made an effort to emulate her positive behavior, I would have been a lot happier and more pleasant to be around.

My stress level would have decreased. My relationships would have been more meaningful. My overall health and wellness would have been better. This example illustrates how we are influenced by the people we surround ourselves with.

Consider who the influencers are in your life. If they are positive, encouraging, and want what's best for you, you're off to a good start. A key ingredient to happiness is surrounding yourself with supportive, loving, happy people. These should be the people closest to you. Ideally, they should be the people you spend the most time with.

However, this isn't always the case when it comes to co-workers and certain family members. That's why it's important to have your positive tribe easily accessible when life is challenging.

A common misconception is that happiness is a destination. It's having a lot of money, a dream house, a fancy car, or traveling to exotic locations. This is similar to believing that you'll be happy when you lose weight.

Imagine that you lose 50 pounds and achieve your weight loss goal. Do you immediately have an abundance of confidence and a perfect, trouble-free life? Of course not! You may have more confidence. You will feel a lot better. Hopefully, you've developed sustainable healthy habits.

The bottom line, just because you're at your happy weight, doesn't mean that challenges evaporate. Happiness begins with your mindset, how you feel about yourself, as well as being grateful for what you have. Other people and possessions (e.g. money) should not define your happiness.

At the height of my corporate career, I was very well paid and finally reached my desired income level. However, my increased salary brought a lot more stress, more time at the office, and less time to do the things I really enjoyed. My health and well-being declined. It turned out my large paycheck did not bring me happiness.

Earning more money may make you happier in the short term. It can reduce stress levels if you've been living paycheck to paycheck. However, according to psychologists, humans quickly adjust to additional wealth.

> **A common misconception is that happiness is a destination.**

Their spending habits increase. This is called "hedonic adaptation."

It's human desire to always want more, based on changing circumstances. Studies show that once a person's basic needs are met, having additional income has little impact on overall happiness. You may have a more expensive house and car but, over time, these things lose their appeal, which creates the desire for something new with the latest bells and whistles, every couple of years.

According to ***Happify,*** a well-being website, 57 percent of Americans say that experiences make them the happiest, especially when they include family and friends, provide a memorable story, are linked to their personal values, and are unusual.

Even if these experiences are not perfect, our brains tend to focus on the positive moments, forgetting the negatives. For example, the airline lost your luggage, but the vacation was outstanding, or your oven broke while cooking your Thanksgiving turkey but the laughs with the family that year were most memorable.

Another study showed that spending money on others, through gift-giving, makes us happier, as does finding ways to give others pleasure. This can include giving of your time.

Being in nature is considered a mood elevator. The combination of natural light and fresh air sends dopamine to the brain, increasing feelings of happiness. Happiness is just one benefit of being in nature. Other health benefits include: improved mental health due to a reduction in stress, increased focus and concentration, a strengthened immune system, decreased blood pressure, and diabetic health benefits.

Outdoor recreation promotes a healthy lifestyle. Walking or biking outdoors can burn from 149 to 372 calories every 30 minutes. The following information, from the National Institutes of Health, Frontiers of Psychology, Nature.com, PLOS ONE, and Semantic Scholar, identify the following nature benefits:

- 10 minutes of gardening or a weekly visit to a public park or garden can alleviate depression.

- 20 minutes of hiking among trees, bird-watching, or doing other nature activities, reduces cortisol, the hormone that causes stress.

- 30 minutes of sitting or walking in a park can lower blood pressure and heart rate.

- 45 minutes of hiking in the mountains results in less fatigue and higher alertness than the same amount of time spent indoors on a treadmill.

- 60 minutes of walking in nature can improve memory and attention span by 20 percent.

Happier people make better decisions, which impact all areas of life. They are more active and make better food choices, resulting in more energy and better sleep. Happier people have lower blood pressure, reduced stress levels, and a stronger immune system. They have more meaningful relationships and are better communicators. They are more supportive, empathetic, and better listeners.

Happier people are more likely to bounce back from a challenge or setback. They look through the lens of a glass half full and consider setbacks as learning experiences. Lastly, happier people are more confident and have a better self-image. They may be a work in progress, but they are confident in their abilities. As a result, they tend to be more successful in business.

Reflection
questions:

1) On a scale of one to ten, how happy do you feel?

2) What is one thing you can do today that will increase your happiness?

3) Who are the happiest people you know? Think about how they live and what they do to maintain their happiness.

_____

_____

_____

_____

_____

CHAPTER 19

GET & GIVE FORGIVENESS

As a child, learning to apologize and ask for forgiveness is a tough lesson. The more difficult lesson is to grant that forgiveness. A playmate broke your favorite toy; you were devastated and angry. You started plotting revenge even though it was an accident. If the perpetrator apologized and asked to be forgiven you may not have been willing, initially.

Fast forward to adulthood. When someone lies to you, you feel betrayed, hurt, and angry. The thought of forgiving that person is unthinkable. You keep replaying the situation over and over in your mind. How could they betray your trust? You can't sleep. It's difficult to focus on anything else.

We get into the same mental turmoil at our own mistakes. A bad financial investment, an error at work, or a poor meal choice makes you chastise yourself for being irresponsible.

The pandemic brought considerable changes to your work and home environments. Working from home made it easy to be less active and led many of us to other unhealthy habits such as the daily happy hour or the family-sized bag of chips for lunch. As a result, you gained a substantial amount of weight, you can't believe how you let yourself go, and you're so disappointed in yourself.

Whatever the situation, forgiveness is the essential key to regaining and maintaining your overall health and wellness.

Forgiveness, by definition, is letting go of resentment, bitterness, anger, or revenge against a person, incident, event, or even yourself. It has nothing to do with the other person, although we often make it all about the other person or situation.

> **Forgiveness has everything to do with your inner healing and restoration of mind, body, and soul.**

It does not mean that we forget what occurred. Forgiveness has everything to do with your inner healing and restoration of mind, body, and soul. When these toxic emotions are not dealt with, they can cause high blood pressure, depression, anxiety, stress, heart disease, and certain types of cancer.

So, how do we release those painful emotions, and forgive?

1) Acknowledge the pain — Validate that you're having the emotion. You're human and entitled to your feelings. You're not a bad person. This is a time to feel your emotions and accept them.

2) Pray — If you're a spiritual person, surrendering to a higher power, through prayer, can be freeing. It can provide hope when you're feeling lost.

3) Meditate — Making time to sit quietly, focusing on your breath or your surroundings, can relieve stress and provide clarity.

4) Journaling — The act of putting pen to paper or typing your thoughts, can also be freeing. I like to call this a good brain dump. Let your thoughts bubble up and ramble if necessary. If your resentment is toward another individual, you can write a letter to them and then burn it or tear it up into tiny pieces to release your emotion.

5) Talk to someone — Talk to a close friend, family member, counselor, coach, or pastor. Sharing with someone who is objective can put things in perspective and provide clarity.

What's most important to remember is forgiveness provides freedom. Releasing toxic emotions enables you to learn, grow, and find peace. Forgiveness is a gift you give to yourself.

Reflection
questions:

1) Who do you need to forgive?

2) What tool will you use to provide that forgiveness?

3) How do you feel when you've granted forgiveness?

CHAPTER 20

BE AUTHENTICALLY YOU

We've all had those moments when we're the outsider. It can happen when you are surrounded by people from different socio-economic, religious, or political backgrounds, or when you were thrown in with "experts" and you had limited knowledge about the topic or skill. These situations make you uncomfortable and fearful of sharing your true self. I was an outsider in my mid 20s when I became an operations manager at a local department store in a predominantly black neighborhood.

I was the minority. I was scared sh?@!%$+! I told myself that no one would take me seriously. I was under-qualified. My people-pleaser saboteur told me I had to bend over backward to make people like me. What I quickly learned is trying to be somebody you're not is a form of self-sabotage.

The only way to earn credibility is to be your true, authentic self. You may not be welcomed with open arms, but you will earn respect by being yourself and taking a genuine interest in others. Be curious, ask questions, and engage in real conversation, not just superficial pleasantries. Genuinely show you care about others and treat people with respect. It took time to earn the respect of the staff, but I did.

Being authentic is liberating, and gives you the freedom to live true to your values and purpose. It gives you the confidence to see yourself for who you truly are and appreciate your uniqueness. This leads to greater happiness, love, and acceptance.

Loving and accepting yourself doesn't mean that you're completely satisfied with every aspect of yourself. It means that you accept your imperfections, recognizing that you're human. Instead of looking at your imperfections as weaknesses, they become learning opportunities, which lead to growth.

Authenticity requires vulnerability. Vulnerability is often considered a sign of weakness. In actuality, vulnerability is a sign of courage. It takes courage to push through the uncomfortable messy parts of vulnerability. It's scary, as it can expose us to judgment and shaming.

As humans, we want to be liked. We want to feel seen, be heard, and know that we have value. When we are rejected, it's defeating. To avoid rejection, shame, blame, and judgment, we may suppress our true selves. We become inauthentic and live a lie, allowing fear of rejection to keep us safe. This destructive behavior can lead to depression, anxiety, isolation, and illness.

Authenticity and vulnerability have everything to do with health and wellness. Allowing ourselves to be vulnerable and authentic is the first step in developing a healthy mindset. We reduce stress by becoming accepting of ourselves, which leads to happiness. Happy people make healthier decisions and are more inclined to bounce back after a setback.

For instance, you may decide that to be your authentic self you need to take a 30-minute walk after dinner while everyone else in your household is engaged with a digital screen. At first, your housemates may be skeptical of your new lifestyle or try to dissuade you from walking. To stay true to yourself and your goals, you will need to stand firm with your decision and gently remind them that this is for you, not for them. After a while, you may find that you have company on your evening strolls. You are no longer the outsider, but the leader!

Making healthy lifestyle changes impacts more than just ourselves, especially if there are multiple people in the same household. Developing healthy habits involves shifts in diet, food preparation, activity, and sleep. If other members of the family are not on board with the changes, tensions can escalate, making success difficult. Having tough conversations involves vulnerability. In this case, it may require courage to ask for what we want. This may feel selfish. However, if the conversation is loving, open, and honest, the other person is more apt to be receptive.

Being vulnerable and authentic may also require making hard decisions about who and what you surround yourself with. If your mental well-being is compromised by negativity and drama, it may be necessary to

> **Allowing ourselves to be vulnerable and authentic is the first step in developing a healthy mindset.**

do some pruning. Cutting back on the constant news feed, being selective about your social media connections, and avoiding gossip in all its forms help strengthen your well-being.

Being your authentic self will free you up to do what is best for you, stay true to your values, and bring your natural gifts to those who need them.

Reflection questions:

1) When have you felt like an outsider?

2) How did you handle the situation?

3) When do you feel you are being your authentic self?

4) When feeling inauthentic, who can you turn to for support?

5) What will your authentic self do this week?
   How will you ask for what you want this week?

CHAPTER 21

BE A WINNING WARRIOR (NOT A WHINING WORRIER)

I recently listened to a coaching conversation regarding "worrier" versus "warrior." A "worrier" is a person in a state of anxiety and uncertainty over actual or potential problems. A "warrior" is a brave or experienced soldier or fighter. Would you describe yourself as a "worrier" or a "warrior"?

When I asked myself this question, my first thought was I am definitely a warrior. However, the more I thought about it, I also saw instances of a worrier. I have a very full schedule with a long list of tasks to complete each day. If I'm not checking off enough tasks, I start to worry that I'm falling behind. This particularly applies if I've overscheduled myself, trying to accomplish too many things in an unrealistic period of time. Sound familiar? I am taking intentional steps to schedule the appropriate time for both tasks and breaks. Time blocking has helped me tremendously and like everyone else, I'm definitely a work in progress.

Worry is a natural part of life. To say you want a worry-free life is completely unrealistic. It's like saying, I want a problem-free life. Problems will arise and our brains will naturally want to solve the problem, and while we puzzle out the solution we imagine all the negative outcomes, we worry.

Worry, if left unattended, can become all-consuming, turning into anxiety and creating stress in the body.

Effects of anxiety on the body include:

1) A sense of doom — a loss of all hope; the worst is yet to come
2) Panic attacks — can cause the heart to race and can simulate a heart attack
3) Depression — can impact all aspects of life
4) Headaches — can often become debilitating, making it difficult to focus
5) Irritability — can impact relationships and work performance
6) Pounding heart — fight or flight response
7) Breathing problems — can resemble an asthma attack
8) Upset stomach — nausea, cramping, vomiting, diarrhea
9) Loss of sex drive
10) Extreme fatigue — wanting to sleep all the time
11) Increase in blood pressure
12) Muscle aches and other pains

Because anxiety is a form of stress, the body reacts to stress similarly. By definition, stress is the body's way of responding to any kind of demand or threat. When our body senses danger, whether it's real or imagined, it goes into "fight-or-flight" mode, otherwise known as the "stress response." The nervous system responds by releasing a flood of stress hormones, including adrenaline and cortisol. You may find your heart beating faster, your muscles tightening, your hands shaking, your blood pressure rising, and your breath quickening.

> **Worry, if left unattended, can become all-consuming, turning into anxiety and creating stress in the body.**

Overall, your senses become sharper. These physical responses increase strength and stamina, speeding up reaction time and enhancing focus. This prepares you to either fight or flee from the danger at hand. Your nervous system cannot distinguish between emotional and physical threats.

Whether you're enraged over an argument with a friend, stressed over a work deadline, or feeling overwhelmed by escalating bills, your body can react just as strongly as if you're facing a true life-or-death situation. The more your emergency stress system is activated, the easier it becomes to trigger, making it harder to shut off.

If you're like many individuals, you may frequently experience high levels of stress. This causes your body to exist in a heightened state of stress most of the time, which can lead to serious health problems, including:

- A compromised immune system, including autoimmune diseases
- Digestive and reproductive problems
- Loss of sex drive
- An increased risk of heart attack and stroke
- Escalating the aging process
- Physical and emotional pain
- Sleep problems
- Skin conditions such as eczema
- Weight gain
- Lack of mental clarity, including the inability to concentrate, forgetfulness, poor judgment, negativity, anxiety, and worry
- Depression or general unhappiness
- Moodiness, irritability, and anger
- Feeling overwhelmed
- Feeling lonely and isolated
- Developing nervous habits, such as nail-biting

If you're experiencing any of these systems, there are solutions. Anxiety and stress are manageable and awareness is the first step in managing stress.

Reflection questions:

1. Are you a worrier or a warrior?

2. When have you felt anxious or stressed?

3. What were your reactions to that anxiety or stress?

SECTION IV

Physical Self-Care

"Take care of your body.
It's the only place you have to live."

Jim Rohn, Entrepreneur

CHAPTER 22

GET GOOD SLEEP

If you're like many individuals, getting a good night's rest is a challenge. After all, there are other priorities that compete for your time: family, kids, work, and social activities, just to name a few. When schedules are very full, sleep is often considered a luxury.

An occasional sleepless night may leave you foggy and irritable. Lack of sleep over a prolonged period can dramatically impact your health and wellness. There is a direct correlation between lack of sleep and weight gain, and a lack of sleep has also been linked to certain types of cancer.

When I was in the corporate retail world, I existed on four to six hours of sleep per night. If we had a major floor reset, a good night's sleep was three hours. On my days off, I tried to catch up on sleep but usually had too many things to do: cleaning, grocery shopping, and errand running. I lived on caffeine and sugary foods for energy. My body craved high fat, high-calorie food. After years of this behavior, I reached my heaviest weight and was depressed, stressed, and burned out. I had stomach, knee, and ankle issues. I would have ended up in the hospital if I had continued at this pace.

A challenge for many parents juggling a full-time career and family time is the need to wind down after the kids go to bed. Your downtime may involve watching TV, taking a warm bath or shower, and reading, and it may take precedence over sleep.

This choice is a double-edged sword. On the one hand, taking time for self-care, relaxing, and making it easier to go to sleep, is a good thing. However, when this wind-down time impacts sleeping time, you're prevented from getting a good night's rest.

Our bodies need between seven to nine hours of sleep per night to repair themselves effectively. An occasional poor night's sleep won't do serious damage. When this pattern is repeated and becomes a habit, it can cause serious damage. Before you roll your eyes and declare that seven to nine hours of sleep each night is ridiculous, check out these scientific facts:

1) Poor sleep can increase appetite due to its effect on hormones that signal hunger and fullness. Ghrelin is released in the stomach, which signals hunger in the brain. Cortisol levels increase, which can also increase appetite and lead to weight gain.

2) Poor sleep can decrease your self-control and decision-making abilities and increase the brain's reaction to food. Sleep deprivation can also increase cravings for high-calorie, high-fat foods. Lack of sleep leads to late-night snacking and larger portion sizes, causing weight gain.

3) Just a few days of poor sleep can cause insulin resistance which is a precursor to both weight gain and type-2 diabetes.

4) Lack of sleep may decrease your exercise motivation, quantity, and intensity. When you're tired, the last thing you want to do is be active.

5) Some studies have shown that poor sleep may decrease your resting metabolic rate (RMR). One contributing factor is that poor sleep may cause muscle loss.

6) Lack of sleep can also deplete your immune system, making it more difficult to fight off illness. Quality sleep is essential to

maintaining or regaining your health and wellness especially if you already have a compromised immune system.

7) When you exercise, especially with weight-bearing activity, your muscles break down. During sleep, muscles get repaired. When sleep-deprived, your muscles do not adequately repair themselves, compromising strength and flexibility.

8) Severe sleep deprivation has symptoms similar to dementia. Lack of sleep impacts mental health and wellbeing. You tend to be forgetful, foggy, and irritable.

If you struggle to get a good night's rest, here are some tips from www. healthline.com you can try:

- Increase bright light exposure during the day. Natural sunlight or bright light during the day helps improve daytime energy and nighttime sleep quality and duration.

- Reduce blue light exposure in the evening. Blue light from electronic devices stimulates the brain. Stop watching TV and turn off bright lights two hours before bedtime. You can install an app on your smartphone that blocks blue light.

- Avoid caffeine late in the day. It lurks in coffee, tea, soda, and chocolate. Caffeine stimulates the nervous system and may stop your body from naturally relaxing at night. You may feel tired, but your brain remains active.

- Reduce irregular or long daytime naps. Taking an extended nap during the day can disrupt your nighttime sleep. Short 10-20 minute power naps shouldn't impact your sleep.

- Sleep and wake at consistent times. Set a sleep schedule. Everyone has different circadian rhythms. If you typically get up early during the week, do your best to maintain your schedule on the weekends. Sleeping late will make it challenging to go to bed at a reasonable time in the evening. Going to bed late will make it difficult to get up early the following morning. It becomes a vicious cycle. In the end, you'll have less quality sleep than if you had gotten up earlier in the morning in the first place.

- Avoid alcohol before sleeping. Although a glass of wine may make you feel sleepy, alcohol is known to cause or increase the symptoms of sleep apnea and snoring. Alcohol impacts normal sleeping rhythms. You may fall asleep quickly, but your sleep quality will be lower.

- Optimize your bedroom environment. Your bedroom should be quiet, dark, and cool.

- Stop eating three hours before bedtime. Eating late in the evening can negatively impact your sleep. Eating a heavy meal right before bedtime can lead to indigestion and poor sleep quality.

- Relax and clear your mind prior to sleep. Turn off the news or anything that over stimulates you. Take a warm bath or shower, listen to relaxing music, read a book, meditate or practice deep breathing.

- Get a comfortable bed, mattress, and pillow. If you awake in the morning with aches and pains, especially in your neck and back, there is a strong possibility that you need a new pillow or mattress.

When I was a child and through my early 30s, I slept like a rock. I could sleep through anything. Unfortunately, I've become a very light sleeper as I reached my mid-30s and through today. I sleep more soundly when I first go to sleep. The slightest movement or noise will wake me up as the night goes on.

If this describes your situation, I feel your pain. It stinks. Over the years, I've found ways to improve my overall rest. I make sure I'm in bed eight to nine hours before getting up. I read a couple of pages or a chapter in a book before turning off the light. Wearing an eye mask and earplugs has helped me tremendously. I also diffuse lavender in a humidifier by my bed. Lavender is just one of the scents that encourage relaxation. Find one that appeals to you.

> There is a direct correlation between lack of sleep and weight gain, and a lack of sleep has also been linked to certain types of cancer.

There are herbal and homeopathic sleep remedies you can pick up at the grocery store. Something as simple as an herbal tea may help you drift off more easily after a difficult day. If you consistently struggle to get good quality sleep, talk to your doctor. They may recommend an over-the-counter solution or prescribe medication for you. Follow your doctor's instructions and notify them of any side effects immediately, as with any prescribed medicine.

Reflection
questions:

1) What gets in your way of getting a good night's rest?

2) What is your sleep and wake schedule?

3) How will you adjust your sleep routine to improve your rest this week?

CHAPTER 23

DRINK MORE WATER

You hear it all the time, "Drink more water!" Our bodies are approximately 60 percent water. The percentage may vary from 45-75 percent, based on age and sex. Water aids in digestion, cleanses the liver and kidneys, improves organ function, hydrates the skin, and improves the immune system by flushing out toxins.

According to the Mayo Clinic, men should consume approximately 15.5 cups of fluid per day (3.7 liters, 124 ounces), and women should drink about 11.5 cups of liquid (2.7 liters, 92 ounces) daily. Before you panic, these recommendations include fluids from water, other beverages, and food. About 20 percent of daily fluid intake usually comes from food, and the rest from beverages other than water. For many individuals, drinking the daily recommended amount of water can be challenging.

Water is the best to maintain overall hydration and wellness, and to make it more palatable, add flavorings, choose seltzers, or infuse your water with herbs, fruit, or vegetables. Cucumber and mint are two of my favorite water enhancers.

Be aware that diet beverages and unsweetened coffee and tea do not have the same hydrating benefits as water. Caffeinated beverages are diuretics that cause dehydration. If you're drinking caffeinated beverages, balance it with a glass of water. Keep that 1:1 beverage to water ratio in mind when sipping your favorite adult beverage, as the alcohol can also dehydrate you.

If you want to **eat** more water, the following juicy fruits and veggies can help you stay hydrated, plus they come packed with nutrients and fiber.

FRUITS	VEGETABLES
Strawberries — 92%	Cucumber — 96%
Watermelon — 92%	Iceberg Lettuce — 96%
Grapefruit — 91%	Celery — 95%
Cantaloupe — 90%	Radish — 95%
Peach — 88%	Zucchini — 95%
Cranberries — 87%	Red Tomatoes — 94%
Orange — 87%	Green Tomatoes — 93%
Pineapple — 87%	Green Cabbage — 92%
Raspberries — 87%	Cauliflower — 92%
Apricot — 86%	Eggplant — 92%
Blueberries — 85%	Sweet Peppers — 92%
Plum 85%	Spinach — 92%
	Broccoli — 91%
	Carrots — 87%

If water consumption is challenging for you, try these simple tips.

1) If plain water isn't appealing, try adding slices of oranges, lemons, limes, or grapefruit and place in your favorite pitcher or Mason jar. Fill with filtered water. Refrigerate for four hours.

2) Always take a water bottle with you when you leave the house.

3) If you forget to drink your water while working, fill your favorite glass or thermos, and keep it on your desk.

4) Set a reminder on your phone to drink your water.

5) Place a water bottle on your bedside table or next to the coffee pot. Drink the bottle first thing when you get up in the morning. Your reward is your cup of coffee (or tea if preferred).

6) Tracking your water is a great way to measure how much you're drinking. Many health apps and fitness devices contain water tracking features.

On average, I drink a gallon of water per day (128 ounces). My consumption does not include six servings of fruits and vegetables. I have a half-gallon (64 ounce) jug sitting on my desk. It has times of the day markers with inspirational sayings. For example, the 8 am marker states, **"Rise and Hydrate!"** The markers show how much water I have consumed. I can quickly tell if I'm getting behind and have to step up my hydration.

Water is the best to maintain overall hydration and wellness.

I do notice that I feel much better physically when I'm consuming more water. My digestion has improved. I'm clear-headed and have more energy. I get fuller faster when I'm drinking a glass of water with my meal.

You may be thinking, *"There is no way I'll consume 128 ounces of water per day. If I manage to choke it down, I'll be in the bathroom all the time. It is not practical!"*

I'm not going to lie; you will be in the bathroom more often. However, once you start fully hydrating your body, you will notice your desire for water increases. I must take a water bottle with me when I leave the house. Otherwise, I will feel parched.

If this is an area of opportunity for you, start small. As discussed in Chapter 4, it takes very small steps, with consistent repetition, to form a habit. Start with four ounce increments (half a cup) and slowly build momentum. You'll be more inclined to stick with your new behavior.

Reflection questions:

1) Where is your water bottle right now?

2) How often do you currently get enough hydration?

3) What can you do this week to increase your water consumption?

CHAPTER 24

EAT BETTER. MOVE MORE.

When it comes to overall health and wellness, diet and exercise each play a big part. Frequently I am asked which one is better for weight loss and weight maintenance.

In terms of weight, you are 80 percent what you eat. If you're trying to lose weight, you will get results if you focus solely on what and how much food you put in your mouth.

Tracking your food intake has been proven to be beneficial to weight loss. Not only does it create awareness of what and how much you're eating, but it shows food patterns and what is keeping you full and satisfied.

Although a popular method for losing weight, counting calories is not as important. First and foremost, no two calories are created equal. Compare an apple and a cookie. Both may have the same calorie content, but the apple has more health benefits. The cookie is likely a highly processed food and loaded with saturated fat. Healthy fats, such as nuts and avocado, may have similar calories to some processed food but have more health benefits.

BUST A MYTH — CARBS ARE UNHEALTHY AND SHOULD BE ELIMINATED FROM THE DIET.

Carbs can be unhealthy if eaten in excess, especially if they are processed carbs found in packaged foods or white bread. Eliminating all carbs from your diet deprives your body of essential nutrients and much-needed energy. Healthy carbs, such as those found in fruits and vegetables, are rich in vitamins and antioxidants, not to mention that they're high in fiber, which aids in digestion. Steel-cut oatmeal helps lower cholesterol and improves heart health. It's also a great energy booster. Choose smart carbs that are unprocessed to get the most out of them.

BUST A MYTH — PEOPLE WITH HIGH CHOLESTEROL SHOULD STAY AWAY FROM HIGH CHOLESTEROL FOODS, ESPECIALLY EGGS.

Foods high in cholesterol do not cause high cholesterol. Foods high in saturated fat cause high cholesterol. Foods high in saturated fat include red meat, processed foods, and fried foods. Although healthy fats, including oils, nuts, and avocados, have many health benefits, our bodies need healthy fats in moderation. Proper portioning is necessary. Eggs are a great source of protein. Unless you have an egg sensitivity or allergy, it is unnecessary to stay away from eggs, even if you have high cholesterol.

So, how does activity fall into the equation? Studies have shown that incorporating activity with a healthy diet leads to 20 percent more weight loss. If you focus on diet alone, your weight loss will eventually plateau. Exercise is essential for maintaining weight loss. According to a recent Consumer Affairs Study, individuals maintaining weight loss averaged 12,000 steps per day. Average weight individuals averaged 9,000 steps per day. The obesity group averaged 6,500 steps per day.

BUST A MYTH — MUSCLE WEIGHS MORE THAN FAT.

A pound of muscle weighs the same amount as a pound of fat. As previously mentioned, lean muscle requires more energy to maintain, increasing resting metabolism. Therefore, individuals with a lower BMI and a higher percentage of lean muscle mass will weigh less. Remember, lean muscle is denser than fat, which is why improving your fitness shrinks your waistline.

IS SITTING THE NEW CANCER?

Exercise often conjures up images of working out at the gym every day or hiring a personal trainer. Both are great options if you enjoy going to the gym or have the means to hire a personal trainer. However, they are not necessary for optimal health.

Rather than imagining your life as a gym rat, think of exercise in terms of moving more throughout your day. If you spend most of your day at a desk or find that you are taking the car to get to the mailbox at the end of your short driveway, it is time to think about how you can get more movement into your life.

For years, research has provided proof of the adverse effects of smoking and its link to cancer. New research suggests that sitting is the new smoking or cancer. If you're skeptical, here are the facts.

According to Dell Dorn of DORN Innovative Healthcare Solutions, the health risks for prolonged sitting include the following:

- Sitting lowers circulation and metabolism. Lack of circulation can lead to blood clots, a higher risk for heart disease, and a greater chance of contracting diabetes. A slower metabolism can cause weight gain.

- There is an increased risk of colon and breast cancer due to prolonged sitting. Studies show a 40 percent decrease in cancer mortality in physically active patients.

- Prolonged sitting can affect mental health, increase fatigue and stress, and lower productivity. You're at a greater risk for depression when you are sedentary.

- Sitting impacts posture and spine health. The muscles that support your back and neck can become weak and stiff. Prolonged sitting can cause chronic lower back pain.

- Our bodies are designed to move. Research states that when we sit for a prolonged period, day after day, our organs begin to shut down. If you work out every day for an hour but are sedentary the remainder of the day, you do more damage to your health than by moving consistently through the day and not having an actual workout. Ideally, you should move every hour.

It is easy to believe that you can't possibly find ways to incorporate movement into your workday if you have a desk job. Here's what I did when I was in the corporate world, tied to my desk for 12-14 hours per day: I made a point of getting up regularly. I went to the restroom farthest away from my desk. If I had a question, instead of directly messaging my team member, I would get up and go to their desk to ask the question. I would take the stairs instead of the elevator whenever possible. On my lunch break, I would take a quick walk around the building.

THE BEST ACTIVITY FOR WEIGHT LOSS

Throughout the years, I've had many individuals ask me what's the best activity for weight loss.

BUST A MYTH — THE BEST TYPE OF ACTIVITY IS CARDIO, AS IT BURNS MORE CALORIES

It's very simple, the best activity for weight loss is the activity you most enjoy. Early birds might enjoy a walk at dawn but cringe at the thought of a 4 o'clock stroll. A night owl might consider an evening yoga practice the best way to unwind from the daily challenges.

As humans, we gravitate toward things that give us pleasure and are easy to do. If we do something difficult, uncomfortable, or just plain unenjoyable, it is not sustainable. We set ourselves up for failure.

Research suggests certain activities produce the most weight loss. According to www.healthline.com, these activities include:

1) **Walking** — It's easy, convenient, and great for beginners. Walking is easier on the joints than running. A brisk walk can be as effective as running, with less stress on the body.

2) **Jogging or Running** — Running is a great way to burn calories. It can help burn visceral fat, commonly known as belly fat. But it can be hard on the joints. Stretching before and after your workout and investing in the right shoes are essential.

3) **Cycling** — A great way to burn calories with less joint stress. Studies have shown that people who cycle regularly have better overall fitness, increased insulin sensitivity, and a lower risk of heart disease, cancer, and death, compared to those who don't cycle regularly. Being properly fitted for a bike is important to avoid lower back, neck, and knee pain. And, wear a helmet; your brain will thank you.

4) **Weight training** — It is imperative to incorporate weight-bearing activity to maintain strong bones and muscle mass. As

we age, we lose muscle mass, women more so than men. Weight training does not have to be done at a gym with equipment. You can use your own body weight as resistance. Yoga and Pilates are great ways to do this, as are planking and push-ups. Yoga is also a great way to relieve stress and improve mindfulness. Resistance bands are easy to use and are great for when you travel. You can also use canned food or bricks for resistance.

5) **Interval training** — This high-intensity training refers to short bursts of intense exercise that alternate with recovery periods and is a great way to build muscle and endurance. Think *Orange Theory* and *CrossFit*. Many gyms have exercise classes with interval training. Because interval training can be intense; it's best to start slow. Listen to your body. You can build up to a complete circuit.

> **If we do something difficult, uncomfortable, or just plain unenjoyable, it is not sustainable. We set ourselves up for failure.**

6) **Swimming** — It's low-impact and is excellent for people with joint pain. It can significantly reduce body fat and improve flexibility.

Alternative activity suggestions include gardening, dancing, Jazzercise, kickboxing, tennis, golf, pickle ball, shopping, painting, and cleaning. Personally, I love vacuuming! It's a great way to increase your step count. It's not strenuous, and the results are immediate (instant gratification). You can blast your favorite music at the same time.

If you take anything away from this chapter, remember this, our bodies are designed to move. If you have a desk job, consider pacing while taking phone calls. Get up and walk around your office or home every hour. At the very least, do a series of stretches every hour. As you move more, not only will you improve your health and flexibility, but you will feel better. The more you move, the better you'll get at losing weight and maintaining your health.

To answer the initial question, "Which is better, diet or exercise for weight reduction and maintenance?" If you want to lose weight, a healthy diet will get results. Incorporating activity is necessary if you want to lose 20 percent more weight and keep it off long term. Your health is a team effort; choose to move and eat good food.

Reflection
question:

1) What will you do today to start your health and wellness journey?

2) What activity are you willing to try this week?

3) How will you record your progress?

_____

_____

_____

_____

_____

CHAPTER 25

UNDERSTAND YOUR FOOD BEHAVIOR

I love food! Food makes me happy. It's hard for me to imagine food as only a source of energy to fuel the body. My Mother, God bless her, was never a huge fan of food. Yes, there were certain foods she enjoyed more than others, such as paté and dark chocolate specifically. Her favorite way to eat was to graze on small portions throughout the day.

She never had a weight problem because she ate like a bird. That might explain why she never enjoyed cooking or sitting down to a big meal. She often sent my dad and me out to dinner. Burger King was one of our favorites.

When I was a child, every holiday and celebration revolved around food. If I had a great report card, "Let's go out for ice cream!" Birthdays and holidays were often celebrated at nice restaurants. I was always gifted with a chocolate Santa or a chocolate bunny at Christmas and Easter. Valentine's Day usually involved a two to four pound box of See's chocolates. And I wonder why I had a weight problem?!

My parents used food to express their love for me. They grew up during the Depression. Food was scarce then, and chocolate and eating out were considered luxuries. Although my parents' intentions were noble, this practice instilled very bad behavior in me. It has taken me years to change my eating behaviors. It was not easy, and there are times when I still struggle. And like most people, even without the idea of food as a reward or celebration, COVID was definitely a challenge. However, I was able to develop sustainable healthy habits and overcome my obsession with food, and so can you.

A common misconception is that building sustainable healthy habits means that you're cured and will never face challenges. Unfortunately, the world is full of challenges. We will never lead a trouble-free life. If you're an emotional eater (like I am), you will always be an emotional eater. It is truly an addiction, but you can manage it.

It's similar to being an alcoholic. Just because you stop drinking and live a sober, free life does not mean that you are no longer an alcoholic. You will always be an alcoholic. The difference is that sober alcoholics have learned to manage their triggers and replace their response of reaching for alcohol with other behaviors.

The same is true for emotional eaters. Emotional eaters find ways to manage their desire to reach for food. When triggered, they find alternative ways of reacting that do not involve food. The desire is still there, but the response has changed.

If you've been unsuccessful in building sustainable healthy habits, you are not alone. Welcome to much of the world's population. If it were easy, everyone would be healthy and at their ideal weight. If you're tired of yo-yo dieting and are ready to make lasting, sustainable changes in your eating behavior, here are some steps to get you started:

1) **Decide to make a change** — The first step is committing to making a change. Anyone can change their eating habits. The challenge is having the right mindset to make a change. If your head is not in the game, you won't be successful. (Refer to Section II on Mindset for applications on how to shift your mindset.)

2) **Find an accountability partner** — Reach out to a friend, family member, or coach to help you stay accountable. Your accountability partner must be objective, supportive, and

willing to lovingly kick you in the butt when needed. Clearly communicate your expectations to your accountability partner. Let them know how they can best support you. Be specific about what you need. They can't read your mind. However, they will appreciate the direction as they will know they are providing you with the support you need.

3) **Start journaling your food** — Tracking what you put in your mouth creates awareness of food patterns, what keeps you full, and highlights triggers. It's easy to forget those small bites you take throughout the day. They all add up.

4) **Recognize when you're using food to feed an emotion** — Awareness is key. Often our reactions are automatic. When we're fully present, we become aware of behavior patterns. (Refer to Chapter 7 for techniques on practicing mindfulness and being present.) Once you determine the emotion driving the desire to reach for food, look for alternatives to feeding this emotion. The great thing about emotions is they are fleeting. Don't tell yourself you can't have the food. That will make you want it more. Wait for five to ten minutes. Go for a walk. Do some stretches. Fold laundry. Play with your dog. Get away from the food. Most likely, you'll forget about reaching for food. After five to ten minutes, ask yourself if you're really hungry and still want food. If you are, have something to eat. If you're not, wait another five minutes. Find something else to keep you occupied. If you

> Emotional eaters find ways to manage their desire to reach for food. When triggered, they find alternative ways of reacting that do not involve food.

desire food after an additional five minutes, have something to eat. Make a healthy choice.

5) **Listen to your body** — Pay attention to how foods and beverages make you feel. If something makes you feel sluggish, bloated, nauseous, etc., it might be time to evaluate if this is something you should be eating. If you have a food sensitivity or allergy, it's time to address it by noticing your reaction when you eat something and when you avoid it.

6) **Portion control** — Invest in a food scale. Keep measuring cups and spoons handy. If you're out to dinner, use your hand as a form of measurement.

PORTION SIZE

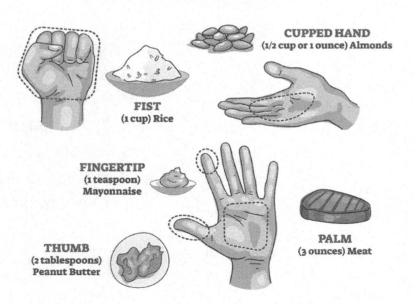

CUPPED HAND
(1/2 cup or 1 ounce) Almonds

FIST
(1 cup) Rice

FINGERTIP
(1 teaspoon)
Mayonnaise

THUMB
(2 tablespoons)
Peanut Butter

PALM
(3 ounces) Meat

Pre-portion snacks and left-overs.

7) **Remove temptations from your house** — If chips and dip are your weakness, don't keep them on hand. I can't keep Girl Scout Cookies in the house. If I do, I will eat an entire sleeve in one sitting. So I now send Girl Scout Cookies to the Troops.

8) **Drink your water** — Always keep your water bottle visible and accessible. Refer to Chapter 23 for guidelines on water consumption.

9) **Allow for indulgences** — If you feel deprived, you're likely to over-indulge. Plan a treat meal. Schedule it, enjoy it, don't feel guilty, and move on! Notice I used the word "treat," not "cheat." Cheat creates a negative image. Treat is more positive.

10) **Manage setbacks** — Life happens. You may have a particularly stressful week, or something unexpected occurs. If this triggers you to over-indulge, own it! Don't beat yourself up. You're human. Most importantly, move on. Lamenting your behavior won't change what has already occurred. It will only make you feel miserable. Bless and release.

Reflection questions:

1) What emotions drive you to reach for food?

2) If you're an emotional eater, what behavior can you do to replace it?

3) What would be your "treat" meal or indulgence?

CHAPTER 26

CHEW ON THIS

As I mentioned, I LOVE food, sweets in particular. I love chocolate cake with chocolate frosting. The more frosting; the better. I love a great hamburger or pizza. I would be remiss if I didn't mention wine; wine pairs well with cheese. Yes, I love cheese too! By now, you're either getting really hungry, or you're wondering what all these things have to do with overall health and wellness.

I'm here to tell you that you can LOVE food and still maintain a healthy weight. You don't have to stick to a Cabbage Soup Diet and lemon water to lose and maintain your weight. I don't believe in eliminating food groups or specific foods. I'm also not a proponent of starvation.

When we deprive ourselves of the foods and beverages we love, we want them more. We may be able to eliminate them for a short time, but eventually, we lose our resolve and cave.

Often, after a prolonged deprivation, we not only cave, but we dive in headfirst. What could have been a managed indulgence now becomes an out-of-control gorge fest. As a result, we feel defeated and often return to our bad habits.

I believe in everything in moderation unless you have an underlying health condition, food sensitivity, or allergy. In these situations, I defer to a healthcare professional. So, with that in mind, let's talk about food and what we should be eating most often.

Consider an average-size plate that was just nine inches in the 1960s. Now, most dinner plates are 10.5 inches, and restaurant plates are even larger. If your plates are super-sized, the salad plate will be more in line with an appropriately sized meal plate to maintain your health. Imagine dividing your plate into four quadrants. Two of those quadrants, or half your plate, should consist of fruits and veggies. One quadrant should consist of lean protein (animal or plant-based, depending on your preference). The final quadrant should consist of whole grains (brown rice, quinoa, barley, and spelt, for example). Assuming you have three meals per day, that would equate to six servings of fruits and veggies, three servings of lean protein, and three servings of whole grains per day.

If you're a snack eater, a combination of fruits, veggies, and lean protein is best. Assuming you have two snacks per day, that would equate to a total of eight servings of fruits and veggies, five servings of lean protein, and three servings of whole grains each day.

The USDA's Dietary Guidelines recommend adults eat between five and thirteen servings of fruits and vegetables per day depending on age, gender, physical activity, and overall health. If you have diabetes, I defer to your health care provider. Depending on your diabetes, you may need to limit fruits and whole grains.

Dairy is an excellent source of calcium and protein, but it has gotten a bad rap recently. Cow's milk has been known to increase inflammation and create digestive issues. If you suffer from chronic respiratory congestion, stomach issues, or inflammation, reducing or eliminating dairy may make a world of difference. Discuss your symptoms with your primary doctor or allergist. If you do not have a sensitivity or allergy to dairy, there are great lower-fat options (fat-free or two percent milk, low-fat string cheese, Greek yogurt, and other healthful choices).

When starting a healthy diet, become accustomed to reading food labels. Many foods, especially processed foods, are high in saturated fat and added sugar. Foods marketed as healthy foods like nutrition bars, low-fat yogurt, and packaged oatmeal can be loaded with sugar, some as high as a candy bar. Many coffee creamers are also high in sugar.

When I started my weight loss journey, I was horrified to learn that my favorite Starbucks beverage contained as much sugar as a piece of cake with frosting. Likewise, the Costco chocolate chip muffins that I loved had as many calories as my pasta dinner. Again, my cranberry juice contained as much sugar as a sweet tea.

> **When we deprive ourselves of the foods and beverages we love, we want them more.**

Saturated fat is found in processed foods such as chips and crackers, meat, dairy products, and seafood. The Dietary Guidelines recommend no more than 10 percent of total calories come from saturated fat.

On the other hand, polyunsaturated fats are healthy fats that can help lower cholesterol. Polyunsaturated fats come from nuts, seeds, vegetable oils, avocado, and fatty fish, such as salmon. Your body needs healthy fats to run efficiently. Therefore, proper portioning of healthy fats is necessary, to avoid overconsumption.

Pay attention to how foods make you feel. Your body is smart. It will tell you when you're feeding it well. As a result, you'll have more energy. Your workouts will be better. Your skin will glow. Your immune system will strengthen. You'll sleep better. You may reduce allergies. As you've learned, If you're trying to lose weight or maintain a healthy weight, a good clean diet is essential.

Reflection
questions/action items:

1) Check the labels on the foods you have in your cupboard. Is there anything you need to purge?

2) This week, journal how the foods you eat make you feel. For example, do you feel satisfied and energized after eating, or do you feel tired and bloated?

3) How many servings of fruit and vegetables did you have today?

_____

_____

_____

_____

_____

CHAPTER 27

CONQUER A WEIGHT LOSS PLATEAU

Imagine that you started a health and wellness journey, and after five months, you have lost 20 pounds. Of course, you're happy to have lost the weight.

However, for the past three weeks, your weight loss has stopped. Your effort has not diminished. You're following a healthy eating plan, you're active, and you average seven to eight hours of sleep per night. Unfortunately, your behavior is not reflected on the scale. You're beyond frustrated! You feel like you've hit a wall. If this resonates with you, you're experiencing a weight loss plateau.

When a person reaches a weight loss plateau, they no longer lose weight, despite following a diet and fitness regimen. Research shows that weight loss plateaus often occur after approximately six months of following a lower-calorie, healthy diet.

When I was on my weight loss journey, I reached a plateau and maintained it for three weeks. I wanted to quit. I was eating very healthy, tracking my meals, walking 15K steps per day, biking 40 miles on the weekends, and hiking twice per week.

Fortunately, I had a coach who was incredibly supportive and encouraging. She reminded me that I had been at my heavier weight for most of my adult life. My body was accustomed to being at a higher weight. It was resisting my weight loss efforts. She encouraged me to stick with it, stating that I would most likely lose several pounds when I moved off the plateau.

If it had not been for my coach, I would have quit. Quitting would have been unfortunate as I had already lost almost 40 pounds. My coach was right. After three weeks my weight finally dropped. I lost over three pounds, an average of one pound per week. Sometimes we have to look at our loss over several weeks to see our progress.

Weight loss plateaus can occur for various reasons:

1. First, your body adapts to your diet and activity.

2. You've become a little loosey-goosey when it comes to your eating plan. For example, you may have stopped tracking your food. You no longer measure and weigh your portions; instead, you're using the eyeball method.

3. Your metabolism slows down due to burning less energy in the same workout you've done for months.

If you find yourself on a plateau, here are some ways to move through them:

•   **Start a food journal if** you're not tracking what you put in your mouth. Journaling your meals, snacks, and beverages can create awareness of patterns and behaviors that sabotage your best efforts. Maybe you're waiting too long between meals or skipping meals altogether. As a result, you're overeating at your next meal. Although your food choices are healthy, your portion sizes may be too large. Too much of a good thing is still too much. It's also easy to forget small bites, licks, and tastes (BLTs) throughout the day.

- **Change what you're eating**. If you're a creature of habit, you may tend to eat the same thing every day. Our bodies become accustomed to what we eat, which can impact our metabolism. Mix things up. You may find your satisfaction level increases.

- **Eat if you're hungry**. Do not take the mentality that less is more. Our bodies require sufficient fuel to run efficiently. If we are not giving our bodies enough fuel, they can store fat for energy. When you're eating the right healthy foods, you may be eating more in volume than before starting your health and wellness journey.

- **Mix up or increase your activity**. As with food, our bodies become accustomed to our activity. For example, imagine that you've taken up cycling. The first time you rode your bike, you managed to ride a mile. Over time, a mile became five miles, then 10 miles. Now you can ride 30 miles on the weekend. Riding five miles now would not burn the same energy you generated when you started cycling. Your stamina and muscle mass have improved. However, your heart rate is lower. You have to ride further or at a higher intensity to get the same workout benefit.

> **Understand that plateaus are temporary.**

- **Reduce your stress**. If you lead a stressful life, your body can overproduce cortisol, leading to weight gain. An overproduction of cortisol can cause cravings for high-fat, high-calorie food. It can also cause weight gain around the abdomen. Refer to Chapter 25 for ways to manage stress and anxiety.

- **Get seven to nine hours of sleep per night**. Lack of sleep also impacts cortisol levels, which can cause weight gain. When you're sleep-deprived, you're less likely to be active. Your body looks for quick energy. You may experience cravings for sugar and carbs. Refer to Chapter 22 for ways to improve sleep.

- **Drink an average of 64-96 ounces of water per day**. Water keeps you hydrated and flushes out toxins that can cause digestive issues and weight gain. Refer to Chapter 23 for tips to stay hydrated.

Weight loss plateaus can be very discouraging and demotivating. They can become the reason to give up, abandoning healthy habits. Understand that *plateaus are temporary.*

Focusing on non-scale victories such as how your clothes fit, your energy level, and how you're sleeping can keep you motivated. Your *"Why"* can also be a strong motivator. For example, why are you trying to get healthy and lose weight? Is it to avoid taking certain medications? Do you want to travel the world after you retire? Is it to enjoy your kids and grandkids as they grow up?

If you find yourself on a plateau, don't give up. Keep doing what you're doing. Get with your coach or accountability partner to help you through it. You've got this!

Reflection
questions:

1) What do you do when you hit a weight loss plateau?

2) What other ways can you stay motivated if you experience a weight loss plateau?

3) Review your **WHY** for weight loss and well-being.

_____

_____

_____

_____

_____

CHAPTER 28

MANAGE YOUR ADDICTIONS

An addiction is when your body craves something that it actually doesn't really need, but has been accustomed to having. Sugar and caffeine are two things that you can live without, but many people would argue that point.

THE SKINNY ON SUGAR

Is sugar really that bad for you? With so much conflicting information on the internet, it's difficult to determine what is fact and what s fiction. Here's the skinny:

In a nutshell, *limited amounts* of processed and refined sugar are not harmful. When consumed in excessive quantities, processed and refined sugar can cause many health problems, including:

- Diabetes
- Obesity
- Heart disease
- High cholesterol
- Certain types of cancer
- Depression

Natural sugar, found in fruits and vegetables, is processed differently in the body from artificial sugar. As a result, fruits and vegetables are high in essential antioxidants and nutrients, so they are recommended for daily consumption. As referenced in Chapter 26, the USDA's Dietary Guidelines recommend adults eat between five to thirteen servings of fruits and vegetables per day depending on age, gender, physical activity, and overall health.

It's important to note that individuals with diabetes or pre-diabetes should consult with their health care professional for their personal recommended sugar guidelines.

Over 70 percent of all processed foods contain sugar, most of which is added sugar. Fruit juice and soda are the primary sources of added sugar. Some fruit juice contains more added sugar than soda. Crazy, right? Especially since fruit juice is marketed as healthy.

Juicing became popular in the 1970s. It's an effective way to increase the number of servings of fruits and veggies you consume in a day. However, it may cause overconsumption of calories.

Juices are more likely to be over-consumed because the brain does not register the same satiety when drinking liquids versus whole food consumption. It's challenging to recognize fullness when drinking liquids. Even if fullness is reached, liquids metabolize more quickly than whole foods. The feeling of fullness is short-lived.

Juices also contain a high natural sugar concentration. Case in point, it takes approximately 13 oranges to make an eight-ounce glass of juice. Would you eat 13 oranges in one sitting? Probably not.

When it comes to potential overconsumption of calories, the same principles apply to smoothies. Additional additives, such as milk, yogurt, and ice cream, can also increase the calorie count.

Approximately 75 percent of Americans eat excessive amounts of sugar. According to www.bornfitness.com, the acceptable amount of added sugar for consumption is:
- 100 calories per day (approx. 25g, 6 tsp) — for women
- 150 calories per day (approx. 38g, 9 tsp) — for men

Those numbers are the equivalent of one regular size Snickers bar or seven to eight Oreo cookies, which is not to encourage you to grab those Snickers or chomp those Oreos. It's to give you a visual of what that pile of sugar looks like. Have you considered what you are adding to your coffee or tea? How much regular soda are you drinking? You should know that a Frappuccino from Starbucks contains **64 grams** of sugar.

Is sugar addictive? Consuming sugar releases opioids and dopamine in our bodies, creating a short-term high and an energy boost. The high eventually turns into fatigue. Sugar, like alcohol, can increase anxiety, stress, and depression. It can also lead to binge eating by serving as a short-term fix for emotional conditions. Research shows that sugar does have addictive properties. However, unlike drugs, the withdrawal symptoms and sensitization are much less.

Sugar by itself does not cause weight gain. For example, one gram of sugar equals four calories. However, you can eat a lot of processed sugar and not feel full, making it easy to over-consume. In contrast, fruits and vegetables containing natural sugar consist of mostly water. They also contain fiber, which increases fullness and satisfaction, making them less likely to be over-consumed.

Bottom line: Be aware of the added sugars in your chosen foods. Everything from tomato sauce to "healthy" juice drinks are loaded with sugar to make them more palatable. The hidden sugar lurking in processed foods will put you over the top.

However, if you enjoy a sugary treat occasionally, go for it! Trying to eliminate processed sugar from your diet is not sustainable long term. It can lead to feelings of deprivation, manifesting into an over-indulgence, which is far more harmful than occasionally having a reasonable portion of your favorite dessert. So, have your cake and eat it too! But, your go-to sweets should be fresh, juicy fruit.

CONSIDER CAFFEINE

According to many studies, moderate caffeine intake has certain health benefits, including lower rates of type 2 diabetes, a lower risk of certain cancers, brain conditions, and liver problems. Caffeine has also been linked to protection against Parkinson's disease. Additional research shows that coffee can improve memory, mood, and energy levels. However, drinking too much caffeine can lead to serious risks. Adverse effects include:

- Increase in blood pressure
- An elevated heart rate
- Shortness of breath or tightness in the chest
- Tremors
- Skin irritations such as hives, eczema, rashes, acne, and severe itching
- Shortened life span
- Headaches/migraines
- Anxiety and panic attacks
- Agitation
- Angry, irritable, bad mood
- Depression
- Delusions or hallucinations
- Numbness in face, hands, or feet
- Restlessness
- Sleeping problems
- Tongue, glands, or throat swelling
- Infertility in young adults
- Muscle pain
- Digestive problems
- Dizziness
- Nausea
- Flu/cold-like symptoms
- Vision problems
- Cold sweats
- Eyes swollen shut
- Fatigue
- Addiction

> **An addiction is when your body craves something that it actually doesn't really need, but has been accustomed to having.**

Some of these effects can intensify when people experience caffeine withdrawal.

One of my former clients had a strong sensitivity to caffeine. She noticed that after consuming caffeinated beverages, particularly coffee, she would get anxious and emotional. It took several months of tracking to realize what was happening. When she stopped drinking coffee, the emotional outbursts went away.

Common sources of caffeine are coffee, tea, soda, energy drinks, supplements, some pain relievers, and chocolate. Understand that while you may not drink coffee, the afternoon chocolate bar is what's perking you up to get through the evening and possibly delaying your sleep.

With conflicting information available, how much caffeine is too much? According to the Mayo Clinic, up to 400 milligrams (mg) of caffeine, a day appears to be safe for most healthy adults. That's roughly the amount of caffeine in four cups of brewed coffee, 10 cans of soda, or two "energy shot" drinks. Some people have little or no reaction to caffeine, while others are strongly affected by much lower amounts.

Keep in mind that the caffeine content in beverages varies widely, especially among energy drinks. In addition, sodas and energy drinks contain sugar, leading to obesity, diabetes, and certain types of cancer. They also contain chemicals that have been linked to cancer if over consumed.

I am an excellent bad example of the adverse effects of too much caffeine. When I was in the corporate world, I existed on caffeine. I drank coffee all day long to stay awake. I was severely sleep-deprived. The coffee was a Band-Aid approach to managing sleep deprivation. After a while, my caffeine consumption backfired. I ended up with stomach problems and acid reflux. Because I often drank coffee late in the afternoon, it impacted my sleep. I was exhausted at 10 pm but could not sleep. As a result, I went to bed too late and averaged four to five hours of sleep per night, contributing to my 65-pound weight gain.

Moderation is your guide to caffeine consumption. If you notice adverse effects, reduce your intake. If your symptoms become severe, it may be necessary to eliminate caffeine consumption. Consult with your doctor.

Reflection questions:

1) What sugar traps do you have in your daily diet?

2) Look through your cupboard and find where sugar is a top ingredient.

3) When you want something sweet, what do you choose?

4) How much caffeine are you consuming daily?

5) What is your body's reaction to the caffeine you are consuming?

6) Is caffeine necessary for you to function?

_____

_____

_____

_____

_____

~

CHAPTER 29

PACE YOUR WEIGHT LOSS

"Slow and steady wins the race" is true for weight loss. Unfortunately, as humans, we want immediate gratification. If we don't see results quickly or don't have a sizable reward, we lose interest. Likewise, if you have a substantial amount of weight to lose, the thought of months and months of dieting is far from appealing. However, if we lose weight slowly, we have a greater chance of keeping the weight off long term.

Consider this; you didn't gain weight overnight. However, it may seem like you did when you look in the mirror one day, and you're horrified by your reflection. You've masked your weight gain by wearing sweats and yoga pants, but now you've got your reality check!

If long-term health is your goal, slow and steady is definitely the way to go. one to two pounds per week is realistic. After that, there will be weeks where you lose a little more or a little less, which is your body's natural way of losing weight.

At some point in your journey, you will reach a plateau. Knowing how to manage a plateau will keep you focused and prevent you from sabotaging your efforts. Refer to Chapter 27 for managing a weight loss plateau.

When there is an important event coming up like a wedding, class reunion, or other special social occasion, people are more likely to look for a quick fix to drop the weight they've been carrying for years to look their best at the event. Drastic diets that limit calories and eliminate food groups may get results in the short term. However, when you return to eating regular portion sizes and incorporating other foods, you gain the weight back.

Losing weight too fast also comes with many health risks, including loss of muscle mass, a decreased metabolism, nutritional deficiencies, gallstones, a higher risk for infection, and a higher risk of a heart attack. Not to mention, you'll likely gain all your weight back and then some.

When you lose weight slowly, you have an opportunity to develop sustainable healthy habits that enable you to keep the weight off long term. Unfortunately, a quick fix does not provide ample time to develop sustainable healthy habits. Habit formation requires repetition to form neural pathways in the brain. With enough repetition, strong neural pathways are formed, instilling positive behavior. Eventually, it becomes second nature. Everyone forms habits at different rates. To say that you'll create a life-long sustainable healthy habit in a few weeks is not impossible but is unlikely. Refer to Chapter 4 on habit formation for more information.

The most impactful way to speed up weight loss is to add or increase activity.

The most impactful way to speed up weight loss is to add or increase activity. As mentioned earlier, you will lose 20 percent more weight when you add activity to your lifestyle. Remember, choose something you enjoy and find other ways to incorporate movement into your day.

How can you incorporate more steps into what you're already doing? Some ideas include parking farther away from your destination, taking a walk at lunchtime, and choosing the stairs instead of the elevator.

If you are consistent and persistent, you will get your desired results. Instead of going for the quick fix, focus on making sustainable lifestyle changes that will reduce stress, allow you to enjoy the journey, and provide long-term health benefits.

Reflection
questions:

1) Have you ever tried a quick-fix diet? How did it go?

2) Using the average of one to two pounds per week, calculate how long it will take to achieve your healthy weight goal.

3) What is one thing you can do today to start your health and wellness journey?

CHAPTER 30

MOVING FORWARD

I hope you've gained insight into how to become your best self. This book aims to create awareness of the pain points in your life that you need to address, which does not mean that you are defective and need fixing. Instead, it means that you are stuck in an unhealthy pattern. Welcome to the majority of the human race. We are all works in progress. Remember, no one is a master of all things; those who appear to have it all together struggle like everyone else.

Creating positive change in your life can and will happen with the right mindset. If you're not there yet, it's okay. However, creating a positive, growth mindset takes time and your commitment. This book is a reference point for you as you move along your wellness journey.

There is absolutely no reason you can't live your happiest, healthiest, and most successful life. You are not too old, and it's not too late. If those influencers in your life are telling you otherwise, they're wrong. There is no limit to what you can do and what you can create. The only limit is your mind.

If you're ready to take a leap of faith and move intentionally towards your best life, I am ready to travel this journey with you. Together, we can do great things.

Let's start by having a conversation. Contact me to schedule a complimentary discovery session. During this 30-minute chat, we'll get to know each other. I'll learn about your life and the challenges you are facing. You'll learn about me and how I help my clients.

> **Creating positive change in your life can and will happen with the right mindset.**

We'll determine if I'm the right fit for you. If we decide to work together, I promise I will show up authentically and support you on your wellness journey. My job is to encourage and challenge you to think beyond your perceived limitations. I'll dare you to dream again. I'll guide you towards your best life. You will do the work, and I will be there to cheer you on each step of the way and offer a loving kick in the butt when you need it. Your best life is waiting. It's time to snatch it!

To book a complimentary 30-minute discovery session, go to:

www.lisahammett.com/book

Feel free to share this book with others. My goal is to help as many people as possible so they can lead their happiest, healthiest, and most successful life.

Lisa Hammett

Lisa Hammett, Success Coaching

P.S. — Let's connect on social media! You can find daily and weekly healthful inspiration and encouragement on all of my platforms.

https://www.linkedin.com/in/lisahammett/
https://www.facebook.com/lisa.a.hammett
https://www.facebook.com/healthylivinglisahammett
https://twitter.com/lisahammett
https://www.instagram.com/lisa.hammett/
https://www.youtube.com/channel/
    UChGQY8WAdQsQnGlFRlIoEbA

ACKNOWLEDGMENTS

Thank you to my amazing friends and colleagues who spent hours reading and providing invaluable feedback on the earliest drafts of my manuscript. I have so much respect and love for all of you — Debbie Ferguson, Tara Gentry, Joani Pepper, Martin Fisher, Joy Booth, Trina D'Elena, Jodie Wallace, and Rich Cavaness.

To my publisher, Susan Friedmann, with Aviva Publishing, thank you for your direction and support in navigating the publishing waters. You made the journey less overwhelming. I value your insight immensely.

Thanks to Kathy Goughenour, founder of Expert VA Training, and Alyssa Berthiaume, Ghostwriter and Writing Guide. Kathy: thank you for introducing me to Aly and for including me in your Virtual Expert conference as a keynote speaker. Aly, thank you for connecting me to Susan Friedmann! I appreciate you both so much. Thank you for your support and encouragement!

To my editor, Jane Maulucci, with The Reactive Voice, thank you for the many hours you spent reviewing and perfecting my manuscript. You are delightful to work with, and I appreciate your sense of humor and support in talking me off the ledge on multiple occasions.

Thanks so much to my super talented and fabulous friend, Kim Guthrie, artist extraordinaire! You took my vision and turned it into the most amazing cover artwork. I appreciate you so much!

To Yael Halpern, my fantastic graphic designer: thank you for creating a beautiful book cover and for spending many hours on layout design. You are truly gifted and a pleasure to work with.

To my super patient and creative web designer and SEO specialist, Ray Liberatore, with Fresh Green Freedom, thank you for creating my beautiful website and for your marketing expertise.

To Art Hoffman, IN-Link Advisors, and his fantastic team, thank you for growing my social media presence and creating raving fans. For the better part of a year, Martin Fisher told me that I should hire you. He was right! Best thing I ever did.

To Kimberley Day, Write and Grow Rich, thank you for your encouragement, support, and for interviewing me on your talk show. You are amazing.

To MarLisa Hollands, The Juicy Life Coach, thank you for allowing me to be a guest speaker in your Magnetic Woman Series. I was so honored to be included with such inspiring women and thought leaders. I appreciate your support and promotion of this book.

To the McKinney Chamber of Commerce and my LINKS networking family, y'all inspire me every week to show up as my very best self. Your enthusiasm and support of my book have been incredible. You truly are family. I am so grateful to you!

To my VTEAM Networking Family, I appreciate your support and encouragement so much.

To my many friends and social media connections who have supported me through the entire book process, from conception to completion, your encouragement and feedback have been invaluable.

To my dear friend, fellow coach, and the most sustaining accountability partner anyone could ask for, Martin Fisher. I could not have gone through this journey without you. Thank you for being my cheerleader, raving fan, supporter, and coach mentor. You are one of the best people I know.

And finally, but first in my heart, to my husband, Tyler Hammett, thank you for putting up with me for 25 years. It has not always been easy. I love you very much. I can't imagine doing life without you.

ABOUT THE AUTHOR

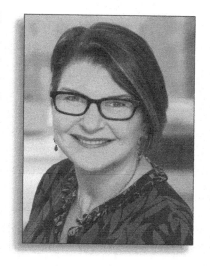

Lisa Hammett was a stressed and completely burned out 26 year retail manager. Then in 2005 she took a leap of faith to follow her passion, reclaim her health, and drop 65 pounds. Upon reaching her wellness goal, she decided to become a service provider, and has spent the last 11 years as a wellness coach, helping thousands of members achieve their health and wellness objectives.

In May of 2020, Lisa launched her Success Coaching practice, to help individuals who were struggling with chronic stress and unhealthy behavior due to the pandemic.

In July of 2021, Lisa joined a global coaching program through HPC — High Performing Coach. During the intensive three-month Launch program, she had several personal breakthroughs that helped her grow personally and professionally. This has enabled Lisa to blend life coaching with her health and wellness experience. Lisa provides her clients with the tools to take charge of their lives, by releasing limiting beliefs that drive unhealthy behavior, and resetting their mindset and actions so they can live their happiest, healthiest, and most successful life.

She is currently working on her Positive Intelligence certification. She offers her clients a six-week Positive Intelligence course to develop their mental fitness so they are better equipped to handle life's challenges with a more positive mindset, and less stress.

Her client success stories include:

- Significant reduction in stress and anxiety by developing mental fitness
- Positive mindset shift
- Improved communication and relationships
- Weight loss
- Improved health
- Building strong confidence
- Development of sustainable healthy habits (mind and body)
- Releasing limiting beliefs and creating space for growth
- Development of a laser focused Vision for goal achievement
- Transition from toxic work environments to careers in alignment with values, passions, and strengths

Lisa's passion is guiding people to achieve their personal and professional goals. She believes that "Everything is possible if your head is in the game." *From Burnout to Best Life* is her first book. She lives in McKinney, Texas, with her husband Tyler and their four-legged kids, Luke and Caymus.